The Family Doctor Speaks:
The Truth About Life

By Robert E. Jackson, Jr., M.D.

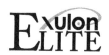

The Family Doctor Speaks: The Truth About Life
by Robert E. Jackson, Jr., M.D.

Printed in the United States of America.
Edited by Xulon Press.

ISBN 9781498499453

www.xulonpress.com

Table of Contents

Introduction

*32 David said to Saul, "Let no one lose heart
on account of this Philistine; your servant will
go and fight him."*

*33 Saul replied, "You are not able to go out
against this Philistine and fight him; you are
only a young man, and he has been a warrior
from his youth."*

*34 But David said to Saul, "Your servant has
been keeping his father's sheep. When a lion
or a bear came and carried off a sheep from
the flock, 35 I went after it, struck it and rescued
the sheep from its mouth. When it turned on
me, I seized it by its hair, struck it and killed
it. 36 Your servant has killed both the lion and
the bear; this uncircumcised Philistine will
be like one of them, because he has defied
the armies of the living God. 37 The LORD who
rescued me from the paw of the lion and the
paw of the bear will rescue me from the hand
of this Philistine."*

*Saul said to David, "Go, and the LORD be with
you." 38 Then Saul dressed David in his own*

tunic. He put a coat of armor on him and a bronze helmet on his head. [39] *David fastened on his sword over the tunic and tried walking around, because he was not used to them.*

"I cannot go in these," he said to Saul, "because I am not used to them." So he took them off. [40] *Then he took his staff in his hand, chose five smooth stones from the stream, put them in the pouch of his shepherd's bag and, with his sling in his hand, approached the Philistine.*

[41] *Meanwhile, the Philistine, with his shield bearer in front of him, kept coming closer to David.* [42] *He looked David over and saw that he was little more than a boy, glowing with health and handsome, and he despised him.* [43] *He said to David, "Am I a dog, that you come at me with sticks?" And the Philistine cursed David by his gods.* [44] *"Come here," he said, "and I'll give your flesh to the birds and the wild animals!"*

[45] *David said to the Philistine, "You come against me with sword and spear and javelin, but I come against you in the name of the* Lord *Almighty, the God of the armies of Israel, whom you have defied.* [46] *This day the* Lord *will deliver you into my hands, and I'll strike you down and cut off your head. This very day I will give the carcasses of the Philistine army to the birds and the wild animals, and the whole world will know that there is a God in Israel.* [47] *All those gathered here will know*

that it is not by sword or spear that the LORD saves; for the battle is the LORD's, and he will give all of you into our hands."

⁴⁸ As the Philistine moved closer to attack him, David ran quickly toward the battle line to meet him. ⁴⁹ Reaching into his bag and taking out a stone, he slung it and struck the Philistine on the forehead. The stone sank into his forehead, and he fell facedown on the ground.

⁵⁰ So David triumphed over the Philistine with a sling and a stone; without a sword in his hand he struck down the Philistine and killed him. ⁵¹ David ran and stood over him. He took hold of the Philistine's sword and drew it from the sheath. After he killed him, he cut off his head with the sword.

When the Philistines saw that their hero was dead, they turned and ran. ⁵² Then the men of Israel and Judah surged forward with a shout and pursued the Philistines to the entrance of Gath and to the gates of Ekron. Their dead were strewn along the Shaaraim road to Gath and Ekron. ⁵³ When the Israelites returned from chasing the Philistines, they plundered their camp. (I Samuel 17:32-53 NIV)

B e bold and courageous, my prolife friend, as David was not afraid of the lion, the bear, or Goliath. Be not afraid of the colossal abortion industry; its foundation is built on lies and falsehood. Pick up your sling and stone and run towards the giant in the name of the Lord Almighty, the God of the armies of Israel whom the murderous abortion industry has defied. Understand clearly that you have only one stone in your sling and that stone is *truth* — the truth that life begins at conception, and that all human life is sacred and deserves to be protected from conception until natural death. Proclaim this truth now and forever until truth strikes down the lying giant opposing God and His precious little ones. When the giant falls to the ground lifeless, the whole world will know there is a God in Israel!!!! Furthermore, when this giant falls, I promise you, it will not be by sword or spear but by divine fiat, in a way none of us would predict, for the battle is truly the Lord's.

Dedication

I dedicate my first book to the people I call heroes of the prolife movement. They are the ones who picketed the only abortion clinic in Spartanburg, S.C., in the 1970s, resulting in its quick closure. They are the pioneers of much of the prolife ministry that has since occurred in Spartanburg County. They are the ones who inspired me and brought me along in my prolife journey.

Josephine Barron
Aileen and George Dawson
Rev. Jack Giddings
Carmella Steele
Rev. Fred Thompson

These courageous defenders of the truth remind me of the sons of Issachar in I Chronicles 12:32. They were "men [and women] who understood the times, with knowledge of what Israel should do."

Acknowledgements

This book would not have been possible without the lessons in life learned from my patients of thirty plus years in residency and medical practice. They are the skeleton of this book while God-given lessons and insights are the sinew and the ligaments.

Thanks to my beloved wife, Carlotta, for being my typist and grammar nazi (my children call her this). She has heard my stories more than anyone, and she still cries. I have to thank my daughter, Hannah, and my wife for conducting the research for the general facts that have been in my mind for decades but needed shoring up and documentation. They love research and do it well. Plus, Hannah took the cover photo and designed the front and back covers. I thank little Ezra Hastings, the sixth child of Matthew and Kim Brooks, for his striking and eye-catching pose on the cover.

Maybe I should apologize to my nine children — or maybe I shouldn't — for dragging them to prolife rallies, marches, and church after church to hear their daddy deliver prolife messages. I am confident my children and my wife could give my main prolife message from memory if called upon. Few things bring me greater pleasure than seeing them engaged in prolife ministries in multiple states. Thank you, children, for your patience and now your own diligence in being "a voice for the voiceless."

My gratitude goes to Alexia Newman for being a strong prolife partner and personal friend since I first met her in

1989. Also, thanks for providing pictures holding wonderful memories from the CPC archives.

Then, my sincerest appreciation goes to Pastor Michael Cloer for his encouragement and example. He allowed me to preach my very first prolife message when he was pastor at Rock Hill Baptist Church in Inman, S.C., in 1985. He introduced me to the prolife rescue community in upstate South Carolina, and he led Pastors for Life in South Carolina for several years. I always have to run to keep up with Pastor Cloer, whether it is in prolife ministry, missions, or just loving Jesus.

Last but not least, thank you, John Richard and Thomas, my special boys. I continue to learn more from you guys than any Bible college education could ever teach me. You have taught me the truth about life more than any other. I love you both to the moon and back.

Endosements

Dr. Robert Jackson is a rare human being with extraordinary skills made even more powerful through his faith in God. His book is bold, scriptural, and loving. His transparency is evident as he shares intimate stories of his family and the struggles he has encountered as a prolife physician. His craftsmanship of words flows from a heart of compassion and a mind of keen understanding. You will be moved as you read this true-life adventure. It is a book that every serious Christian should read.

James Rudy Gray, President and Editor of *The Baptist Courier* and Courier Publishing

While knowing this author for over 30 years, I was not surprised that *The Family Doctor Speaks: The Truth About Life* is unlike anything I have ever read on this subject. With his Biblical worldview as his standard, using his medical knowledge, his godly wisdom, and his decades of experience, he exposes the lies of the abortion industry. However, it is not harsh or judgmental, but compassionate and caring. His passion for saving life is always softened by his love for the hurting. I found myself smiling and at times weeping. These are not stale stories off the newswire, but real testimonies of real people. This should be required reading for every high school graduate and every parent. As a pastor, I want every staff member and church leader to have this book as a frequently used resource.

Dr. Michael Cloer, Pastor
Englewood Baptist Church
Rocky Mount, North Carolina

There are some people that you know when you meet them you will be lifelong friends. That was the case when I met Dr. Robert Jackson, and for over 25 years this has been the case. I have learned so much from this brother and friend in Christ! I have seen him in good times and in the struggles of life, and in them all his faith has never wavered. He has been steady, and he has trusted in the promises of the Word!

This is what makes his book so incredibly special! He has walked this journey of prolife ministry. He has answered many of the questions that plague our nation regarding life and, as you will see, he answered the call when it was time to take his commitment to the next level and be a spokesman for the prolife ministry.

This is a book that once you begin it, you will not want to put it down. You will be immersed in the pilgrimage of this man who loves Jesus, his wife and family, others, and the nations.

Alexia Newman, Director
Carolina Pregnancy Center
Spartanburg, South Carolina

It is my great joy and privilege to recommend this wonderful book for your reading. I have personally known Dr. Robert Jackson for over six years as his pastor and close friend. These amazing God-stories are representative of the great adventure he and his wife Carlotta and their family have traveled. I believe these kinds of experiences happen in Doc's life because his life is surrendered to the Lord, and he offers himself so willingly to be a vessel used by God. Dr. Robert Jackson is one of the foremost voices and advocates for the prolife message. He has lived it on every level, and been used from the pulpit to the pew in the lives of many people. I would recommend any pastor to have him come and speak, as few can, on this most important subject. This book will enlighten and enhance your life of faith and deepen your love for God. It will also create a hunger in your heart to live a life more open to God interventions. Sit back and let the family doctor bless you and challenge you in his own words as he tells these true encounters from his own faith journey.

Dr. Hank Williams
Senior Pastor, Boiling Springs First Baptist Church
Boiling Springs, South Carolina

Foreword

*T*he *Family Doctor Speaks: The Truth About Life,* as the
title implies, is not a book about the horrors of abortion.
It is a book about the hallowed and precious gift of life. The
stories are not about fictional people with made up lives inter-
acting in an imaginary world. Every compelling, page turning
story has been lifted from a life lived in the service of others.
Dr. Robert Jackson's primary passion in life is life itself. Next
to his love and devotion for God, his lifelong love affair with
his wife Carlotta, and his special love for their nine children,
Robert's passion is life. His heart beats to give every unborn
beating heart the opportunity to live, to laugh, and to love
for a lifetime.

As you read these incredible stories, you will laugh, you
will cry, and you will shout out loud for joy at the miracles God
has done and continues to do. Some of these stories are incredibly personal, and not particularly easy for Robert to share. But
through the pain, the passion, the joy, and the praise, you will
experience the grace, mercy, and ultimately the redeeming love
of our heavenly Father. *The Family Doctor Speaks* is a book
filled with Scripture calling each one of us to examine our own
lives in light of the love of life God has revealed to us. In many
places you will be challenged by the hard questions, such as,
"What is the measure of a culture? Do we measure a culture by
how we treat those who are wealthy or famous or powerful,
or do we measure a culture by how we treat those who are the
weakest and infirm and powerless?" God answers that question
in I Corinthians 1:26-29, "For consider your calling, brethren,

that there were not many wise according to the flesh, not many mighty, not many noble; but God has chosen the foolish things of the world to shame the wise, and God has chosen the weak things of the world to shame the things which are strong, and the base things of the world, and the despised, God has chosen the things that are not, that He might nullify the things that are, that no man should boast before God."

As you read, you will be shocked, amazed, inspired, and most all you will be reminded what God can do through the life and family of one very good man. You see, I am fully qualified to talk about Robert's life as one who pours himself into others. He has been my friend, my mentor, my advisor, my counselor, and my most trusted family doctor for almost 30 years. I have lived many of these stories, observing how he and his family have weathered the storms of life while fighting every day for the sanctity of life. I watched his children grow into the amazing, spirit-filled, God-honoring adults they are today and how most of them now have families of their own who are carrying on the legacy of life.

I have benefited from Robert's wisdom, his passion for life, and his devotion to God. The years he has poured all those things into my life now pour forth from the pages of this book in story after story of God's grace. You see, what begins as a collection of stories about life shared by a family doctor, a husband, and a father with a passion for life ends as one continuous story of the love our heavenly Father has for each one of us. Truly, when you have read and savored every story, every page in this book, you will join David as he says, "I praise you, for I am fearfully and wonderfully made! Wonderful are your works; my soul knows it very well" (Psalm 139:14).

He must increase; I must decrease.
Dr. Tony Beam
Vice-President for Student Life and Christian Worldview
North Greenville University
Christ Makes the Difference!

Prologue

After I finished castigating my overweight, diabetic patient for his noncompliant, overindulgent lifestyle (overeating, smoking, carousing, noncompliance with medication) for probably the tenth time, he looked at me with a twinkle in his eyes and asked, "Doc, is that your best advice?"

Thinking we were finally getting somewhere, I replied, "Yes, sir, that is my best advice."

He paused a moment contemplatively, and then he asked, "How much would you charge me for your second best advice?" We both laughed, him more than me.

Doctors constantly dispense advice; some of which is ignored, and most of which, we hope, is heeded. Sadly, we know a significant percentage of prescriptions we write are never filled, for a variety of reasons. We give advice regarding blood pressure, blood sugar, cholesterol, weight control, headaches, asthma, etc. Like the family priest/counselor, we are even called upon to intervene in family squabbles, give recommendations on child rearing, and provide marriage counseling.

Christian doctors have an even higher calling to speak the truth of the gospel into the lives of their patients regarding a whole host of issues as time and opportunity permit. We understand that God's Word speaks to the issues of life in a pertinent and powerful way. "The Word of God is living and active and sharper than any two-edged sword, and piercing as far as the division of soul and spirit, of both joints and marrow, and able to judge the thoughts and intentions of the heart," (Hebrews 4:12). We would be remiss if we did not share the truth of God's Word with our patients who are hurting or confused.

For example, just last week I counseled with Terri and Mark for forty-five minutes concerning an entire married life of unforgiveness. Neither one of them knew how to appropriately deal with conflict in their marriage. Each time a conflict occurred, both of them brought up every offense the other had committed in all their previous years of marriage. I shared with them Psalm 103:12, "As far as the east is from the west, so far has He removed our transgressions from us," and Isaiah 43:25b, "And I will not remember your sins." I carefully pointed out to both of them that God never forgets, but this means He does not keep a ledger book because all of our sins have been placed under the blood of Jesus and completely washed away. I also pointed out they were guilty of keeping a ledger book against one another and were equally guilty of unforgiveness.

Of course, we talked about a whole host of other issues as well. I finished by challenging them to write down a list of everything each knew he or she had personally done to offend the other partner. They were to go through the list item-by-item, asking forgiveness of the other partner. They were then to write 1 John 1:9 over the entire list, which says, "If we confess our sins, He is faithful and just to forgive us and to cleanse us of all unrighteousness." We would meet again in two weeks to see how they did on their homework assignment.

Paul told the Ephesians they should be "speaking the truth in love," (Ephesians 4:15) which is a hard balancing act for all of us. Only Jesus perfectly balanced speaking the truth in love, and we all know where that got Him–crucified by His enemies and abandoned by His friends. You and I must seek the grace of God in this responsibility of speaking truth into the lives of others and doing so with genuine Christian love. I will readily confess that I do not get it right all of the time, but I am working on it and daily practicing the art of truth-speaking from a heart of love.

After thirty plus years of practicing medicine, my patients know I love them. I try to be delicate when I speak biblical truth into their lives. Most folks accept it because they know who I am and for Whom and what I stand. They may not do the right thing, but they listen politely and respectfully. I always appreciate that. Some people don't want to hear a biblical perspective. I respect that, too. I treat them politely and respectfully, knowing they will need me another day. They may be open to the truth then, just like my patient David.

David was an alcoholic and an angry man for most of his adult life. I treated him for depression and chronic pain due to multiple surgeries. His friends called him an atheist, although he denied this designation. He was so angry he was denied services at multiple pharmacies due to angry outbursts. My staff could hardly put up with him. I prayed for him every Friday for three years and told him so. He told me not to bother.

He would not listen to any biblical advice for his issues, which were numerous, until one day he came to me and apologized for an angry outburst the previous month. The apology was entirely out of character for him. "David, if I could make an observation, I suspect the spirit of God is really at work in your life. I tell my Sunday School class that you can tell the character of a Christian man by what he does when he is confronted with his sin. Does he slough it off? Or does he man up, confess it, and make things right? It is not like you to confess wrongdoing and apologize. I perceive God is at work in your heart."

He looked at the floor, then confessed, "Doc, I hate to admit it, but I think you are right."

"Well, I think it is time for you and me to meet somewhere for breakfast so we can talk about life."

"Doc, I would love to do that, but I'm afraid."

"Afraid of what?"

"I'm afraid I'll cry. I don't want to cry in front of you."

"David, both men and women cry in front of me every day. Sometimes I cry, too."

"Well, I'll think about it."

"By the way you know what today is, don't you?"

"Yeah, yeah. It's Friday. It's the day you pray for me. Maybe God is listening to you after all."

In this book are similar anecdotal experiences of speaking the truth in love. Some will make you laugh, some will make you cry, and some will make you angry. I trust they will encourage and challenge you to do the same, especially in the area of the prolife struggle confronting all of us. Each story is true. All of the characters are real. The names and circumstances have been changed a bit in some of the stories to protect the innocent–or the guilty, as the case may be. If a last name has been provided, then those individuals have given me permission to provide their names and stories intact.

————— ◆ — ⋯◆⋯ — ◆ —————

If I were to invite all of you to meet me in my hometown of Manning, South Carolina, we would all travel there by different routes and by different modes of transportation, and we would all arrive at different times. Eventually, we would all get there. In like manner, all genuine believers have a prolife journey. Yours may not look like mine. The journeys of your friend, neighbor, and fellow church member may not look like yours. This book will describe my prolife journey from a medical student with a vague notion that abortion was not right to becoming a strong prolife advocate. This journey took eight years. I suggest we all extend grace to one another and allow God to be unique in each of our lives, in each of our prolife pilgrimages. The only thing I consider unacceptable for a believer is not being willing to take the journey, not traveling with others on the prolife pilgrimage.

My responsibility as a prolife physician is to educate and to motivate. The purpose of this book is to teach you about the fundamentals of this issue and to challenge you to become an advocate for unborn children and their moms. I don't want you to just be informed; I want you to be involved. I suggest you should do the same, especially for the next generation — your children and grandchildren. Who will teach them if you don't? This book will share with you interesting and intriguing stopping off places on my prolife journey and the lessons I have learned in life. You will also meet some fascinating people and hear some amazing stories from the country doctor's rusty, dusty scrapbook.

Chapter One

My Prolife Pilgrimage

To get to my hometown of Manning, South Carolina, I drive down country roads shadowed by oak trees draped with Spanish moss and lined by deep, dark swamps. They seem to take me far away from "the madding crowd" and toward a happy and safe place. Manning was where everyone truly knew everyone else. Once someone wrote a letter to my grandmother, Mrs. Anne Land; it was addressed to Mrs. Earth but, yes, the postman still knew exactly to whom it should go. In Manning, we could dial a wrong number and still talk for fifteen minutes. Don't laugh — I've done it! Manning was an idyllic place where every child should grow up. Manning was where life seemed to pass by slowly. At least, that's what I thought as a young boy.

Roe v. Wade became the law of the land when I was a senior in high school. I didn't even know it. It didn't touch my world as a teenager in my little hometown of Manning, probably because the war in Vietnam was ending. The Vietnam War and Watergate dominated the news my senior year in high school, but sports and academics dominated my little world, certainly not current events. If this Supreme Court decision legalizing abortion on demand was discussed, I never heard it. At least I don't remember such discussions, and I think I would. Throughout college, abortion continued to be a non-issue for me. I never talked about it, nor did I hear others debate or struggle with the issue in any way.

This suddenly changed when I appeared at the Medical University of Charleston for my medical school interview in 1977. Unbeknownst to little, ignorant me, I was about to be interviewed by a gentleman who was a department chairman in the school and had been married five times and divorced five times, and who was dating a girl who was a ward secretary at the VA hospital. He was like the woman at the well in reverse. The interview also included a female who was an instructor in the obstetrics and gynecology department, as well as the director of the abortion clinic in Charleston. She presided over many thousands of abortions during her tenure there. Like *Sleepless in Seattle*, I was clueless in Charleston.

As they interviewed me, they asked me all the superficial, perfunctory questions that interviewers usually ask, but it didn't take them long to figure out I was an evangelical Christian. I don't remember how, but the truth just came out. I guess the saying is true, "When you squeeze a lemon, you get lemon juice, and when you squeeze an evangelical Christian, you get Jesus." It ought to be so, anyway. The interviewers looked at each other, and then they looked at me. There was a long, pregnant pause before they asked me this question, "Let's just suppose your best friend came to you and confided in you he had gotten his girlfriend pregnant. He has come to you for advice. What would you advise him to do?"

I considered this a moment while I pulled out of my pea-sized brain and pea-sized wisdom the following answer, "Well, I don't know that advising them to get married would necessarily cement their relationship together. I suppose I should talk to them about adoption. That would be something they should consider. I know some good pastoral counselors I could refer them to. Of course, I would continue to be a close friend to him and encourage him in every way I could." Then I stopped. I had nothing more to say.

We all sat there, continuing to look at each other, until the female doctor finally decided to ask, "Well, what about abortion?"

I almost exploded with a subdued shout, "Good gracious, no! Why would you kill the baby when the baby hasn't done anything wrong?" Remember, I was oblivious to whom I was speaking, and remember I had never debated the topic with anyone.

She responded, "Why not?"

I answered again with a question, "Why would you add a whole lifetime of remorse and guilt to this young woman when her life is already complicated by an unplanned pregnancy?"

She looked at me momentarily with bewilderment in her eyes; then she said, "The medical research does not show that abortion causes a lifetime of remorse and guilt." (Also, remember this is 1977, only four years after *Roe v. Wade*, which is not much time for vast amounts of research regarding abortion consequences.)

Respectfully, I replied, "Ma'am, guilt is a function of the Spirit of God, and when you involve yourself in a terrible thing like abortion, I promise you, you are going to have guilt and remorse for the rest of your life!" Now here I was, a punk college kid trying to get into medical school, and I'm disputing with a woman who's an instructor in a medical school about medical research and telling her that I don't believe the medical research.

Well, she sat back in her chair, stroked her chin as if she had a beard, and pondered my statement for a moment before she conceded, "Robert, I just happen to believe you are right." The meeting was over. I was dismissed. The rest is history, because somehow they accepted me into medical school.

Three years later I found myself in the obstetrics course required of all medical students. The instructor was the same doctor who presided over the abortion clinic. Usually our classes were rather raucous, filled with questions, answers, and interchange between the doctors and the students, but not this time. As we sat in one particular lecture, cold, dead silence filled the room. Why? She was addressing the various abortion techniques and describing to us what she called "therapeutic abortion." In other words, she was teaching us how to kill unborn babies.

It just so happened my chair was right underneath her lectern. Before I proceed, let me explain something to you. In medicine, doctors do not perform surgery unless they have clear surgical indications. To clarify, a surgeon obviously does not want to operate on someone unless it is medically necessary. Otherwise, the physician could set himself up for litigation and embarrassment.

> *In other words, she was teaching us how to kill unborn babies.*

After she finished her lecture, she asked, "Are there any questions?"

The room remained silent, but there on the front row was this long-necked, big-eared, red-headed student who didn't know any better than to raise his hand and ask, "Well, ma'am, what exactly are the surgical indications for these so-called therapeutic abortions?"

Well, that silent class got colder, deader, and more silent. She leaned over the lectern and with cold malice in her voice, she bored a hole through my head and said, "Robert, there are none and we will not discuss it anymore."

She then turned and quickly stalked out the door. I wanted to turn to the class and say, "I rest my case," but I resisted. You understand that in America, unborn babies can be aborted for any reason throughout the nine months of pregnancy. That is why the only surgical indications are $300 cash, and that the mother doesn't want to be pregnant.

Despite these brief episodes of sounding like a prolife expert, I still did not have in my mind or in my heart any clearly defined prolife perspective, nor was I a prolife advocate. I just knew down deep in my heart that abortion was not good or right. Nevertheless, if you had asked me, "Robert, why are you opposed to abortion?" I could not have articulated for you any well thought out answer. All I could have said to you was, "Well, I just don't think it's right," just like most right-thinking evangelical Christian folks. However, I was on a prolife pilgrimage. I just didn't know it yet.

After medical school, I attended the family practice residency program in Spartanburg, South Carolina. I married Carlotta Watson, the eldest and best-looking daughter of a southern-fried Baptist pastor, and we began family practice in earnest, having the first child of nine in 1984. (She is the queen of my life and I love her desperately!!)

While in residency, I picked up the recently written book *The Right to Live; The Right to Die* by C. Everett Koop, a pediatric surgeon whom President Ronald Reagan tapped in 1982 to be Surgeon General, a position in which he served until 1989.[1] In general, I remember reading his viewpoints on life–there is no such thing as a life not worth living, and everyone has a right to live. He contended that if we ever decide there is a life not worth living then we have put our feet on a very slippery slope, a very slippery ethical slope of moral relativism that does not end until we hit a moral quagmire at the bottom that includes abortion, euthanasia, and infanticide. I read and pondered this book deeply for a summer. Then two significant events pushed me further along on my prolife journey.

One event began and ended in the emergency room where I took care of a patient in the middle of a miscarriage. She was about three months along. Usually, when a woman has a miscarriage this early, what is delivered is barely recognizable. It just looks like blood and tissue, but on this particular day something extraordinary happened. As I assisted this woman in her distress, she delivered into my right hand a twelve-week baby. It was still in an intact bag of water, the amniotic sac, and the baby was alive, perfectly formed and moving in that bag of water. I had never seen anything like it. The baby was about three quarters the length of my hand. What I carefully and tenderly held was a miniature human being. He stayed there for probably five to six seconds until suddenly the bag of water broke, and the little baby shriveled and died right there in my hand. The mother saw all of this, and she began to weep uncontrollably. Her cries drew from me a great big sob. I held the baby over to the nurse and asked, "What is that?"

With a big question in her eyes, she declared, "Why, Doctor Jackson, that's a baby!"

I nodded with sorrow, "Yeah, that's what I thought." That's what I thought, all right. I mean, "it" looked like a baby, moved like a baby, and died like a baby—right there in my hand, and we all saw the plain and simple truth!

During my research on abortion in upstate South Carolina, I learned when most women in South Carolina, and around the country for that matter, went to the abortion clinics to obtain abortions. I learned babies were about eight-to-twelve weeks of gestation when most of these abortions were performed. I learned that in the nearby town of Greenville, abortionists performed between 3,182 to 3,905 abortions per year at three different abortion clinics between 1980 and 1986.[2] I remembered all that "learning" as I considered the twelve-week gestation baby in my hands, and I dropped my head in horror and grief.

The second event occurred while I was on a pediatrics rotation. A woman in town abandoned her newborn child, a premature infant. Brought to the hospital in the paste-board box in which he was found, he was the smallest child (at one pound, nine ounces) resuscitated successfully at Spartanburg Regional Hospital at that time. The nurses in the neonatal intensive care unit named him Nathan. As a black child, he was so hypoxic (deficient in oxygen) that upon his arrival he was as black as coal, shriveled, and barely alive. Only a miracle brought him to the hospital alive, where it was my privilege to be a participant in his care.

We put a catheter in his umbilical artery. We put him on a ventilator. We put him on oxygen and then commenced to care for him at the cost of many thousands of dollars per day for many, many months. He experienced every conceivable complication from sepsis to meningitis to pneumonia to ischemic bowel. His list of problems got longer and longer but he lived; he survived every single one of them. Months passed, but he finally graduated from the intensive care unit weighing just over four pounds, eight ounces; later, he went home with foster parents. All of us marveled to see him leave the hospital. We had all grown to love Nathan as we prayed many prayers over his tiny little body!

When he was two years old, I saw Nathan in the pediatric clinic. He was a very "bad" two-year old boy, but as I looked at him, I thought I was seeing my own long-lost child because I had invested so much time and so many sleepless nights monitoring his blood gases, pondering his white blood count, and examining his chest x-rays in the middle of the night. I dropped to my knees and exclaimed, "Nathan! Nathan!" I wanted to say, "Come to Daddy!" but I knew he wouldn't understand. Neither Nathan nor his foster parents knew who I was; nevertheless, I wanted to hug him and squeeze him. He just crawled into his foster mom's lap with a quizzical expression that asked, "Who are you?"

By looking at Nathan's size and shape, his little hands and feet, and other features, we doctors figured he was approximately twenty-two weeks gestation when he showed up in the intensive care unit. At the same time he arrived, so did a pregnant woman who was also about twenty-two weeks pregnant. Her baby had hydrocephalus; in lay terms, "water on the brain." A specialist talked to her, evaluated her, and told her that the very best thing for her to do was to have an abortion. She didn't want any part of it, but she was literally brow beaten into an abortion by the specialist, a neurosurgeon. With a great deal of reluctance and weeping, she agreed to it.

I happened to be on call the night the medication inducing labor was to be given to her, a prostaglandin suppository. They asked me to give her the medication. I politely refused, saying, "I'm sorry. I cannot do that."

Well, my refusal required a third-year obstetric resident to come in from his home at midnight to give the medication, which, of course, he did not want to do. His indignant and irate response was, "No, I'm sorry. You have to give the medication. I am not driving in just to give that suppository." (You see how being obedient to God and standing up for your convictions is often not a simple thing. It sometimes complicates the lives of others, arousing their ire and misunderstanding.)

He and I went back and forth with our "I'm sorry, but I'm not," and, "Oh, yes, you are," for a while until an uproar commenced on the fifth floor labor and delivery of our hospital. Our disagreement quickly escalated from him to the resident above him to the attending surgeon to the surgeon above him, and so I found myself in the eye of the storm. They threatened to kick me out of residency and to fire me from my job.

To be honest, I was pretty calm because I was resolved in my heart; giving an abortifacient was just something I could not do even if they thought the baby's life was not worth living. I could not and would not violate my conscience. They were in a fizz, a big fizz, until the situation finally got to the top, to the chairman of the obstetric department, Dr. Ruble — God bless him. Dr. Ruble arrived, assessed the situation, and decreed, "You cannot violate this man's conscience." He called the third year resident and informed him, "You will come in and give the medication." He did, but he was not happy about it.

During the night the woman experienced violent contractions induced by the prostaglandin suppository, and she prematurely delivered her baby the next morning. Born alive, he was wrapped in a cold, wet towel, placed in a separate room from his mother, and left to die all alone. I just happened to be walking through and saw him lying, exposed, in a metal basin. I can still hear his weak, dying cries. I heard his mother wailing all up and down the fifth floor of the hospital. I walked by the nurses' station, where three nurses wept and held one another. I said to myself, "What is wrong with this situation? This is a labor and delivery floor. These women are supposed to be happy. This is a fun place. If aborting this child was such a good thing for this woman, why are these folks not happy?"

All of this transpired on the exact same floor where we took Nathan, also twenty-two weeks gestation and whose mother had rejected him, and ushered him into a room only twenty steps further down the hall, and spent thousands of dollars a day to resuscitate him and preserve his life. Why the double standard? Why was one child's life deemed worthy of saving and preserving and another child's life deemed not worth living? Why such hypocrisy? These questions pounded my head day and night.

This first phase of my prolife pilgrimage was about to end. Shortly thereafter, a brand new radio station, WLFJ, began broadcasting in May 1983 from Greenville, South Carolina. I was driving home in my burgundy, 1977 Monte Carlo. As I drove, those questions continued to plague me while I listened to WLFJ. Soon a public service announcement came on. A granddaughter in the future asked her grandfather,

35

"Granddaddy, do you mean to tell me that in the 70s and 80s it was legal to kill little babies before they were born?"

The grandfather responded, "Yes, yes, darling, that's true."

She pondered for a moment, and then obviously quite agitated, she said, "You mean, Granddaddy, they could take little babies from their mothers' wombs and kill them and that was legal?"

"Yes, that was true."

Silence hung in the air; then she asked, "Well, Granddaddy, what did you do to help put a stop to it?" Again, silence, a long silence... then that was the end of the public service announcement because Granddaddy had nothing to say. Granddaddy hadn't done a thing to help put a stop to abortion.

Neither had I. In that moment, the Holy Spirit of God put a spiritual dagger into my heart because I was an American citizen, I was a born-again Christian, and I was a medical doctor. I knew better than anybody what grew in the mother's womb. I was the one who looked at the ultrasounds of the pregnant women for whom I cared, and yet I was the one who had never done anything practical to help stop even one abortion. I was brokenhearted! I drove my car about a mile and a half further down the road, pulled up to my first little house, laid my head on the steering wheel and wept. I covenanted together with God that as long as I had breath in my body I would protest abortion, and I would do all I could to end abortion in America. I have been faithful to that covenant. I have sponsored rallies. I have prayed at abortion clinics. I have debated congressmen. I helped start four crisis pregnancy centers. I write my legislators. I speak in churches and at prolife fundraising banquets. I teach at the volunteer and counselor trainings at our local CPC. I counsel women and men in my office. I even spent a few days in jail in the 1980s after blocking the entrance to an abortion clinic. I had a great prison ministry!

I tell you the above not to brag on myself, but to communicate to you the brokenness and conviction propelling me into action and to challenge us all to be diligent in doing all we can to right this horrible travesty perpetrated upon the unborn, their parents, extended family, our country, and the church by abortion on demand. When faced with the atrocities of the Nazi regime, Dietrich Bonhoeffer proclaimed, "Silence in the face of evil is itself evil: God will not hold us guiltless. Not to speak is to speak. Not to act is to act."[3] I determined in my heart that I would speak up, not for myself, but for the unborn children of America. My journey had begun!

Chapter Two

The Bottom Line

While in my third year of medical school in the middle of an obstetrics rotation, a fellow medical student engaged me in a rather heated debate regarding the morality of the abortion procedures taught in a lecture earlier in the day. One of my classmates, who happened to be one of the top students in my class, ended the discussion when he looked at me and said, "I would just as soon step on a cockroach as perform an abortion procedure." Completely floored by the callousness of this statement, I had no further comeback. I couldn't believe that this highly intelligent, academically gifted friend had no more moral compunction about performing an abortion procedure in which the life of an unborn human being would be snuffed out than to step on the ever-present cockroaches that invaded every nook and cranny of Charleston, South Carolina.

Consider the following excerpt from an article entitled, "Woman Seeks Custody of Dead Fetus" in the *Spartanburg Herald* newspaper published May 18, 1989.

> The mother of a pregnant girl killed in an April head-on collision near Campobello wants legal custody of the dead fetus so she can file a wrongful death suit on the fetus's behalf. Greer attorney David M. Rogers filed a petition last Thursday in Spartanburg

County Probate Court so Helen J. Gibbs of Mill Spring, N.C., could become personal representative of the unborn boy killed with his mother in the April 14 head-on collision. The accident, believed caused by a game of dare between two drivers, also killed a Campobello woman whose parents have filed a $2 million wrongful death suit. If Mrs. Gibbs is appointed, Rogers said he plans to file a wrongful death suit on the dead fetus's behalf. A hearing is scheduled before Probate Judge Raymond C. Eubanks Jr. at 10 a.m. June 13. Rogers said that in South Carolina there have been a "handful" of cases where someone becomes the personal representative of a dead fetus. A person appointed representative has the authority to bring lawsuits and settle estate claims, he said. "You don't see that very often," Rogers said, adding that several of the previous cases involve fetuses killed in car accidents. To file such a petition, Rogers said, the fetus must be "viable," meaning it could have lived outside the womb. The Probate Court petition states that because the child was 8 1/2 months pregnant [article should have read gestation] it could have survived outside the womb. "If the child is killed or injured before birth, an action can be maintained," Rogers said. "We're bringing the action because of the death of the child."[1]

I remembered this accident, as it occurred a few miles from where I lived at the time. I sat pondering this whole story because I realized this teenage girl could have driven to Atlanta earlier on the day of April 14th and paid an abortionist to terminate the life of her baby. This would have been perfectly legal. Yet here was a grandmother trying to get custody of a dead fetus in order to file a "wrongful death suit on the fetus's behalf." This custody battle was eventually dropped in a settlement of the case.[2]

Nevertheless, the controversy continues to surface as babies are killed in the womb by criminal behavior in case after case across the country. Thankfully, as of March 2015, thirty-eight states have fetal homicide laws with the majority giving full-coverage to the unborn victim "under names such as the Fetal Protection Act, the Preborn Victims of Violence Act and the Unborn Victim of Violence Act."[3]

However, in some states such as Colorado, the battle still rages over crimes committed against an unborn baby. For example, let us look at a more recent event in Colorado. Everyone would admit being horrified by the case of a pregnant woman, Michelle Wilkins, going to the home of another woman, Dynel Lane, on March 18, 2015, to purchase baby clothes advertised on Craigslist. Lane was accused of brutally attacking Wilkins and removing her baby from her womb. Wilkins survived, but the baby did not. Because an autopsy revealed the baby had not breathed outside of the womb, under Colorado law there could be no murder charge, only a charge of unlawful termination of a pregnancy.[4]

As one can see, Roe v. Wade leads to bizarre and unjust applications of the law. While in one state, Lane could be charged with murder, but in another she could not. It is difficult to live in a country

> *Roe v. Wade leads to bizarre and unjust applications of the law.*

full of double standards and hypocrisy. Christians must strive to live as God-fearing, right-thinking people with a single Biblically informed moral standard.

Another dramatic incident drove this truth home when a patient came to see me. She was a beautiful, blond-headed girl, a cheerleader, and a senior student at a Spartanburg High School planning to attend medical school after college in order to be a pediatrician. Academically qualified, she could have made this dream come true.

It was my difficult task that day to tell her she had a positive pregnancy test. Breathing a silent prayer, I opened the door and walked in. There she sat, a movie star face with big blue eyes staring at me. My mind immediately flew back to her five-year old well-baby check up when she sat on that same exam table with blond curls and patent leather shoes, nervously waiting for the doctor, knowing she would later receive her baby shots. Now she anxiously awaited the results of a pregnancy test. Not hopeful and expectant like my married patients, she desperately prayed for a negative test; such was not to be the case. My, how things change.

I knew this young lady quite well, having cared for her most of her seventeen years. I also knew that the news I held in my hand would change her life forever. With much compassion and concern and understanding the potential for a significant blow to this family, I delicately revealed the positive test. I could not control my tears as I watched the weight of her choices descend upon her. For what seemed like an eternity, we wept together as her mother sat stone-faced. Her mother did not even offer her daughter any solace. Eventually, I found the words to encourage both mom and daughter. Holding both of her hands in mine, I looked the daughter straight in the eyes. "You know this changes dramatically the direction of your life, but it doesn't ruin your life because God is a sovereign God who will give you grace. You will be a good mother. You will raise this child to be a God-fearing child of the King," I assured her.

When I finished, her mother exploded. She had had all she could take, and she declared emphatically, "She is not going to have this child, and tomorrow we are going to Greenville to the abortion clinic. She will abort this child." The daughter looked at her mom, then to me, and once again to her mom, all the while sobbing even more uncontrollably.

I pleaded, "Mama, you can't do that! It would violate all of your deepest personal convictions." Her mother then stormed out of the exam room without another word and left the office. I looked at that beautiful, blond haired girl, and I said, "You need to go home with your mama, but appeal to your daddy, because he is a good man." I knew her father was a deacon in a church while her mother taught Sunday School in that same church.

What happened in that exam room that day? How could this mother, a lifelong Sunday School teacher, suddenly jettison her convictions and sacrifice her own grandchild on the altar of her daughter's academic pursuits? What happened in that room is what happens to many of us when we are caught in social dilemmas. We allow our circumstances to dictate our theology rather than allowing our theology to dictate our response to difficult circumstances.

We become victims of situational ethics. This mother was cut adrift in a sea of moral relativism. She lost her biblical mooring. The circumstances of her life so overwhelmed her that she was willing to agree to legally sanctioned child murder to avoid public humiliation amongst her peers

> *We allow our circumstances to dictate our theology rather than allowing our theology to dictate our response to difficult circumstances.*

and to allow her daughter to pursue her academic goals.

We must all understand the world on the outside looks in askance at those of us in the church, wondering how we will respond to the vagaries of life. Whenever we are hypocritical or practice double standards, like this mom, this behavior is all they need to discard Biblical Christianity, saying in their hearts, "I knew it would never work. Just look at those Christians. They are such hypocrites."

When I prayed at the abortion clinic, fully half of the cars that came into the parking lot had some kind of church logo on them. The abortion doctors claimed if it weren't for the church people, they couldn't stay open. According to a study by the Guttmacher Institute, over half of abortion patients in 2014 reported an affiliation with a Christian religion–"24% were Catholic, 17% were mainline Protestant, and 13% were evangelical Protestant. 8% identified with some other religion."[5]

O God, forgive us for our hypocrisy. We, the church, have blood on our hands as well.

It is imperative if we claim to be a people of the Book that we live lives consistent with Biblical standards. If we claim that life is sacred and created in the image of God, then how can we discard the lives of innocent unborn children simply because our daughters and granddaughters find themselves pregnant at inconvenient times?

I am not insensitive to the difficult circumstances in which young women find themselves, but we must remember if that which grows in the mother's womb is a human being created in

there is no circumstance, no matter how desperate, that justifies the killing of an innocent, unborn human being.

the image of God, then there is no circumstance, no matter how desperate, that justifies the killing of an innocent, unborn human being. I understand those circumstances — no boyfriend, no husband, no insurance, loss of a college scholarship, certain illnesses that complicate a pregnancy, and fading dreams — but one cannot justify the killing of an unborn child on these or any other altar. I've dealt with every single one of these circumstances, and some of them are indeed heart breaking and heart wrenching, but again I tell you on the authority of God's Word there is no circumstance that justifies taking an innocent life. You and I must be convinced of this truth. If we aren't, then we can never be staunch, consistent prolife advocates. We will flinch when the fire is hot or the circumstances seemingly too difficult.

We must be convinced in our heart of hearts that Jesus can meet every need of the human heart, even that pregnant teenage girl who is unwed and without adequate social support. Otherwise, we will flinch and look away in her hour of deepest need. We must have faith enough in Jesus' supernatural ability to meet her needs through you and me (i.e. the church). We must look her straight in the eye and assert confidently, "Having this baby is the right thing to do, and we will stand with you all the way, through thick and thin. Jesus is Jehovah Jireh, the Lord who provides. He will provide everything you need. Trust in Him and do right!" Although the right thing may be hard in the short run, it is always best in the long run and it holds no regrets.

What exactly is the bottom line in all of this prolife discussion? The bottom line is the answer to one question - what grows in the mother's womb? I'll let Dr. John C. Willke, an obstetrician and gynecologist and past president of National Right to Life answer the question.

> *The bottom line is the answer to one question—what grows in the mother's womb?*

> This is the question that must first be considered, pondered, discussed, and finally, answered. It cannot be brushed aside or ignored. It must be faced and met honestly. Upon its answer hinges the entire abortion

question, as all other considerations pale to insignificance when compared with it. In a sense, nothing else really matters. If what is growing within the mother is not human life, if it is just a piece of tissue — a glob of protoplasm — then it deserves little respect or consideration, and the primary concern should be the mother's physical and mental health, her social well-being, and, at times, even her convenience.[7]

Is that which grows in the mother's womb a potential human being or a human being with enormous potential? If that which grows in the mother's womb is a potential human being, then abortion is a nonissue. There is no reason to be emotionally distraught. There is no need to write a congressman. There is no need for crisis pregnancy centers because the moral significance of an abortion procedure is no different than the moral significance of an appendectomy or removing a gall bladder. However, if that which grows in the mother's womb is a human being with enormous potential, created in the image of God, special in the economy of God, one for whom the very Son of God died on a cruel Roman cross, then none of us should lay our head on our pillow at night until we have satisfied our conscience that we have done all within our personal power to put a stop to what amounts to the wholesale slaughter of innocent unborn human beings.

This is the bottom line — the unborn baby is an innocent living human being whose life is sacred. Therefore, no circumstance justifies the killing of innocent human life. All social dilemmas, no matter how difficult or desperate, pale into insignificance compared to the value of the life of an unborn child.

I am happy to report that this young woman's story did not end that day in my office. Seventeen years later she returned to the exact same exam room with her seventeen-year old son. It happened to be his birthday, and he needed a sports physical. He was about six foot two inches tall, big and strapping even at his age. He was all knees and elbows with a large lantern jaw. I could tell he would be one of those men who would have to shave twice a day. It was obvious that his mama did not go to medical school, nor did her academic dreams come true. However, I could tell she was extremely proud of her son.

After I examined him, she came back into the exam room, looked at me with tears in her eyes, and asked, "Dr. Jackson, do you remember?" whereupon we both suddenly began to tear up. I immediately recalled the titanic spiritual battle that took place in that exact same exam room seventeen years previously for the life of her now seventeen-year old son. She said, "Dr. Jackson, thank you. Thank you for helping me do what was right. All of my dreams did not come true, but my dream of being a mama one day — that did come true. I am so proud of my boy, and I'll tell you one other thing — his grandmother loves him to death!" While we hugged each other and wept yet again, albeit seventeen years later, I wondered what her son thought about this entire scene, this time a scene of celebration.

Chapter Three

The Hard Cases

The crisis pregnancy center in Rock Hill, South Carolina called one day and asked if I would speak to a woman named Lisa who had an issue that was beyond their expertise. "Of course," I said. Lisa and I eventually became close friends, even though we never met personally.

I prayed, picked up the phone, and prepared myself for what probably would be a difficult story. I was right. Lisa Williams was about thirty weeks pregnant. Although she was a Christian woman, she was not married. She had recently been diagnosed with an aneurysm in her brain. Her obstetrician had told her emphatically she would die in childbirth because of the aneurysm, and abortion was her only option. Because of her Christian belief system, she completely opposed an abortion. Devoted to her unborn child, she had committed to maintaining the pregnancy. What should my advice be to this woman who had a seventeen year-old son, an unplanned pregnancy, and an absent father?

After quietly listening to her story and consoling Lisa, I offered my best advice, "Miss Lisa, you will have to be like Jesus to your unborn child. You

> *you will have to be like Jesus to your unborn child.*

have to be willing to give your life to give life to your child, if necessary, as Jesus did for us. I cannot promise you that you will survive. In fact, I cannot promise that to any given woman in any given pregnancy. I can only promise you will have a clear conscience before God, and you will know you made the right choice in giving life to your child. I can certainly promise you if you have an abortion you will live the rest of your life with regret, knowing you participated in the killing of your unborn child. Furthermore, your doctor cannot guarantee you will have complications from the aneurysm as he seems to be so confidently asserting at this point in time."

She cried many tears on the phone. We prayed together, and she left me saying she would discuss it further with her pastor. I warned her in advance that her physician would say she was foolish if she elected to maintain the pregnancy.

One month later she called to say, "I am being cared for by a specialist at the Medical University of Charleston, South Carolina because my local obstetrician declined to care for me. He referred me to a specialist at the Medical University." In my opinion, her doctor made the right decision in referring her since she was a high-risk pregnancy. She also made the right choice. She chose to give life to her child, despite the inherent risk to herself.

Shortly thereafter, she delivered a healthy baby boy without any complications to herself or to the child. She named him Royalty. Two years later she had the aneurysm repaired surgically by a specialist at a hospital in Washington, D.C. For years she called me every two to three months to update me on Royalty's status and her own, and she sent me a Christmas card with their picture on it. I kept it on my desk for a long time to remind me to pray for them. With a grateful heart I often look at their picture and shout, "Glory!"

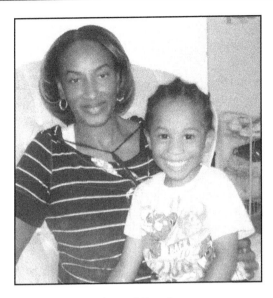

Lisa and Royalty

To repeat, it is always best to do the right thing, even in difficult circumstances. A situation may be embarrassing, frightening, or even life threatening, but God honors those who choose life and choose to do the right thing.

People come to me all the time, and they say, "Yeah, Doc, we hear what you're saying, but be for real. What about those hard cases? What about rape and incest? What about the handicapped children?" They often agree with me that using abortion as a form of birth control is completely unacceptable; nevertheless, they still struggle with what I, and others, call the "hard cases."

Well, let's be honest with one another. In the United States, statistics reveal that 98% of abortions are what we call "convenience" abortions, which means that the abortion procedure is being used for birth

> *98% of abortions are what we call "convenience" abortions.*

control, i.e., the mother does not consider it convenient to be pregnant at that time. Consider the following:

> The actual percentages of U.S. abortions in "hard cases" are estimated as follows: in cases of rape, 0.3%; in cases of incest, 0.03%; in cases of risk to maternal life, 0.1%; in cases of risk to maternal health, 0.8%; and in cases of fetal health issues, 0.5%. About 98.3% of abortions in the United States are elective, including socio- economic reasons or for birth control.[1]

In Exodus 4, we find the biblical account of Moses and the burning bush. Moses had just spent forty years in the back desert of Midian squeezing sand between his toes and listening to sheep bleat when God appeared suddenly to him in a burning bush. God gave Moses an ultimatum, saying, "Go down to Egypt land and tell ole' pharaoh to let my people go."

What did Moses say? "But, but, but God, I can't do that. I st-st-stutter" (according to Robert Jackson's paraphrase of v. 10).

What was God's response? In Exodus 4:11-12 God rebutted, "Who has made man's mouth? Or who makes him dumb or deaf, or seeing or blind? Is it not I, the Lord? Now then go, and I, even I, will be with your mouth, and teach you what you are to say." Now I don't begin to pretend to understand why God makes some people whole and some people handicapped, but God doesn't apologize to anybody. He assumes full responsibility for those who are deaf, blind, mute, or handicapped in any other fashion. I don't know why God has given my beautiful bride and me two special needs boys, but I do not expect God to apologize to me or to explain himself away. Furthermore, if anyone suggests to me that those two precious boys' lives are not worth living or are in some way inferior, then I'm going to give them a righteous fat lip!!

Not one, but two–two special needs children in the Jackson household. Yep, God saw fit to send two our way. We think we have an inkling of an understanding of, "Why?" but we'll probably ask for more clarification when we see Him face to face. In the meantime, we care for these two every single day. When we joke with extended family about the size of our family, we ask them, "Which one(s) would you want us to send back?" No one ever answers that question, although we do wonder sometimes if they think Thomas, our Downs child, or maybe John Richard, our "who knows what" child should be sent back.

John Richard, named for my two brothers, entered God's world on September 28, 1993, the same day as his mom's birthday. He was past due, so I took my wife to the hospital on a Thursday morning, where a nurse began a Pitocin drip to induce labor. Carlotta unapologetically likes her epidurals (although some of the children arrived without one), so at some point in the morning she received an epidural. However, we discovered the baby was in a breech position. As a family physician I had delivered all of our babies, but I decided to consult an obstetrician on this one. When the doctor arrived, he decided my experienced wife could deliver this baby normally without a C-section, so he ordered the epidural to be turned off and the Pitocin increased. That sounded painful to me even thou I wasn't the one in labor. I knew what she was thinking without asking. I was right.

Nevertheless, she faced the coming hours with remarkable pluck, and in short order delivered a second Jackson boy (but sixth child). I watched the doctor hand a very blue and lax baby over to the nurse, but after a few seconds he pinked up and appeared mostly normal. I say "mostly" because one ear looked like it was folded in half, his head wasn't exactly nice and round, and he had extra fingers on both hands. His initial Apgar score was low, but the second one was about an eight or nine out of ten. (We don't remember exactly.) Thankfully, his ear soon plumped out to normal size and his extra boneless, little fingers were removed. Upon leaving for home, the nurse told Carlotta she might want to keep an extra eye on "this one" as he looked a tad blue around the mouth in the nursery; plus, she gave us a machine to monitor his breathing.

During the next month as John Richard declined in health, my wife took him to every doctor known to man. Doctors tested, poked, prodded, x-rayed and scanned him from head to toe. One neurologist suspected seizure activity because his eyes rolled back in his head when he was feeding. A cardiologist said to "look for something else," despite two or three minor "holes" in his heart. Oxygen was delivered to the house, and we held blow-by oxygen to his nose when he was sleeping (which meant no sleep for us). Technicians checked his oxygen levels at the house, at the hospital, and in offices; the levels varied just enough to tell us he needed a little oxygen but not enough to give us a diagnosis. Whenever he tried to feed from a bottle, he grew fatigued, his eyes rolled back in his head, and he literally passed out. Nevertheless, no one could tell us what was wrong until an almost fatal day.

John Richard developed a cold, causing him to seem weaker than usual. Carlotta took him to a local hospital where doctors ran more tests, including arterial blood gases. They checked it twice because after the first attempt the blood gases were so low they thought they had drawn blood from a vein. Confident they had hit an artery the second time, the doctors and respiratory therapists were stunned at how low John Richard's blood oxygen levels were. Despite this, they sent us home holding blow-by oxygen to his nose, because again nothing pointed to a specific diagnosis. I guess because my wife and I are medical people, they thought we could manage.

We sat perplexed on our back porch that day holding oxygen to his nose, and we prayed over him and plotted our next move. I called the pediatric heart clinic doctors who came from Charlotte, North Carolina to Spartanburg once a month to provide specialty care, since we did not have a pediatric cardiologist. I told the very understanding doctor on call that I was trying not to be an overwrought doctor-daddy, but I knew there was something desperately wrong with my baby boy. I just couldn't put my finger on a diagnosis. He immediately said, "Bring your baby to the ER in Charlotte. I will be glad to see him." Our fearful and confused hearts soared with gratefulness at that invitation. After consulting with him by phone, we decided to disperse our five other children to close friends and head for the Carolina Medical Center in Charlotte. No one knew the answer to John Richard's problem, but we were not going to sit at home one more night holding oxygen to his nose.

We arrived around midnight and checked our son in to the emergency room; then they transferred him to the pediatric intensive care unit while we moved in to a facility for families of patients. Three hours later they called to tell us that John Richard had experienced a respiratory arrest, had to be intubated, and put on a respirator. We looked at each other, confident the Holy Spirit had nudged us to leave home just in time to probably save our son's life. We could have been home when he arrested. Even now I am moved to tears contemplating what could have happened that night if we had stayed home and he had suffered a respiratory arrest at home in the middle of the night. We are both medically trained, but performing CPR on our own four-week old son would be more than I can imagine.

The next day a pediatric pulmonologist looked down John Richard's airway with a bronchoscope and diagnosed largyngotracheomalacia. Three days later, they placed a tracheotomy in his airway. Three weeks later, John Richard was transferred to one of our local hospitals, then sent home after another week with a feeding tube, a tracheostomy, and oxygen to the trach.

We thought he was on the way to recovery, getting bigger, and growing up, but for two more months he did not prosper. He failed to gain weight and continued to be pale and bluish in color. We finally heard a pediatric pulmonologist in Greenville had just purchased a new, tiny bronchoscope that could examine further down into the bronchii of the lungs. She diagnosed malacia of John Richard's bronchii in addition to the trachea and larynx, for which reason she put him on a bi-pap machine, a type of respirator that forces positive air pressure into the lungs with each breath, thereby dilating the airways deep into his lungs.

After four long months we finally had a diagnosis of laryngotracheobronchomalacia, which means a floppiness of the cartilage of the entire airway down into the lungs, causing the airway to collapse down upon itself and cutting off the flow of oxygen. How do you like that one? We sounded so intelligent just saying the word, laryngotracheobronchomalacia. The bi-pap machine blew oxygen into John Richard's airway under pressure, thereby keeping it from collapsing for the first time in four months.

The good news — this problem could be outgrown. As a child's body grows, so does the diameter of the airway. Therefore, John Richard just had to grow physically bigger. With proper oxygenation for the first time since birth, he began to do just that. The bad news — we had a mini-intensive care unit in our home in addition to nurses around the clock for a few weeks, then incrementally decreasing their hours over the next few months. The respirator, tube feedings, and trach required constant care, and when the nurses weren't at the house, it was my wife, our other children, and myself left to provide this care. The children, the oldest being nine, learned how to tube feed him, take him on and off oxygen, and even suction his trach. Even the two year old ran to us and reported, "Sucsh," which meant John Richard's trach needed to be suctioned.

Life as we knew it came to a halt. No more piano lessons, no more violin lessons, no more gymnastics, no more attending church together as a family. My wife resigned all of her church and extracurricular responsibilities. I went to work and back. We traded off attending church. We traded off buying groceries. I brought home many takeout meals. Occasionally, we had a wonderful respiratory therapist who gave us respite during the day and who even went on a Florida vacation with us–driving us down, washing our clothes, cooking our food, and caring for John Richard's tracheostomy while we took the children to Disney World. James Splawn, we will never forget. You blessed our family beyond words.

When John Richard was ten months of age, the feeding tube had been long gone, and the respirator finally vanished from our home, but so did the nurses. This meant John Richard and his crib were moved to our bedroom where we continued to care for his trach, which had to be attached to a humidifier system every night. That long blue tubing hung along his bed, and every night fluid would collect in the bend and start gurgling. Carlotta or I would roll over and tell the other, "It's your turn to empty it."

Significantly, without the respirator he could now go anywhere with us. We began to live life again, including taking John Richard to church. My wife took him up into the choir loft during choir practice. Remember, he still had a tracheostomy, which had to be suctioned constantly, so up on the stage went a double stroller holding him and his suction equipment. Without fail we also carried around an extra trach appliance in case the current one became so stopped up we couldn't suction it out, requiring us to remove it in an emergency. This happened one time.

John Richard vomited and an abundance of vomit went down his trach, making it impossible to suction it all out. Thankfully, I was home and able to exchange the trachs quickly enough. I tried to look calm and professional for my wife's benefit, but it was still a heart-pounding event!

Think about this and be thankful when your babies and grandbabies scream their hearts out. For most of John Richard's first eighteen months, he was a silent baby. You see, when a person has a tracheostomy, no air can pass through the larynx for vocalization. We only heard mucus sounds in his trach, including when he screwed up his little face and looked like he was crying, but we couldn't hear him. We could not hear him! There was no sound! He would only strain and become red in the face.

Once while we were changing his trach, he managed to force air up his airway and past his vocal cords. He suddenly began to cry lustily like a normal baby. Except for the day he was born, we had never heard him cry. He was almost a year old! Carlotta and I looked at each other, and we began to cry ourselves, realizing what we had been missing. How can one cry over missing a baby's cry? Aren't we strange people?

Life began to resume some sort of normalcy, including another pregnancy. Yep, being pregnant was pretty normal for us in those days. This was number seven. Ten days after our next son arrived on March 13, 1995, we were back in the intensive care unit in Greenville, South Carolina for another joyous occasion. John Richard had grown so much he no longer needed his tracheostomy, so the surgeons removed it and repaired his trachea. Oh, happy day! Only those who are familiar with a tracheostomy will ever know what a happy day it was. Truly, life returned to normal. Well, is life really normal with seven children? We consistently had new normals (and still do), but we loved it.

At the time of this writing, John Richard is twenty-two years old, a handsome, beloved member of our family, our church, and our circle. He has the mind of a four year old. We don't know why; they told us something probably happened in utero, not from a lack of oxygen during the first months. This means our "normal" life included years of multiple doctor visits and eleven years of therapies–occupational, speech, and physical. Additionally, he has a severe hearing loss, so he wears bilateral hearing aids and has speech deficiencies. Nevertheless, we all *love* John Richard, his blond hair, and those huge, deep dimples.

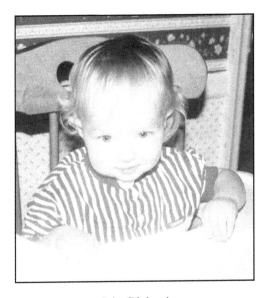

John Richard

What do parents and grandparents say when they find out they are expecting? It doesn't matter whether "it" is a girl or a boy as long as "it" is healthy. Of course, we all know what we mean by that statement, but what if the baby isn't healthy?

Jeremiah 1:4-5 states, "The word of the Lord came to me saying, 'Before I formed you in the womb, I knew you. Before you were born, I set you apart; I appointed you as prophet to the nations.'" This passage makes it plain that before Jeremiah was a gleam in his daddy's eye, God had a plan for his life. Before the foundation of the world was laid, before any footsteps were heard in the halls of history, before he was conceived in his mother's womb, God knew all about Jeremiah and had a special plan for his life. God had set him apart to be a prophet to the nations. I submit to the reader, very respectfully, that you and I are no less valuable to God than Jeremiah. Your life and mine and the life of every child conceived since Adam and Eve is sacred in the economy of God, having been created in the image of God.

I believe God has a special plan for every child, including John Richard, and that plan was conceived in the heart of God before the foundation of the world. Every abortion abruptly and prematurely terminates the divine, predetermined

> *I believe God has a special plan for every child, including John Richard, and that plan was conceived in the heart of God before the foundation of the world.*

plan of God for a child, who is sacred and special in the eternal plan of the Heavenly Father, who looks over the ramparts of heaven with a broken, grieving heart to behold what we are allowing to happen with His precious little ones.

This begs the question—who are we to abort the plan of God? Who are we to intervene and terminate the plan of God? Who are we to arrogate to ourselves the right to assume that just because some children are born with handicaps that their lives will be less in quality than others who are born seemingly whole? Only God can see into the future and can foreknow the quality of a person's life. We may not arrogate to ourselves the right to be the judge and jury in advance of the quality of a person's life.

> *We may not arrogate to ourselves the right to be the judge and jury in advance of the quality of a person's life.*

It is dangerous when we depart from the sanctity of human life ethic and place our feet on the slippery slope of the quality of life ethic. Once we begin to assess that some lives are not worth living because of their handicaps, there is no stopping until we hit the bottom of that ethical slope.

——— · ━ ··◆··· ━ · ━———

Our local crisis pregnancy center in Spartanburg called to ask me to speak with Becky Rice, a schoolteacher from Gaffney, South Carolina. Once again, I replied, "Of course." Later, she presented to my office where she informed me that a prenatal test revealed a genetic defect called Trisomy 18 in her unborn child. These children are born severely mentally handicapped, usually with little to no brain, and often die before or within hours after birth. She wrote her story down for me, so here are her words.

BECKY

I was forty-four years old. I had one daughter who was recently married, one daughter about to graduate from high school, one son thirteen years old, and a sick husband who was unable to work. I was devastated when I went to the doctor and learned I was pregnant. I thought I was going through "the change." The OB doctor told me I needed to have several tests, and one test confirmed the baby boy had Trisomy 18. This meant the baby would either need several operations after birth or he could even be stillborn. A vortex of feelings, emotions, and questions enveloped me. I went to my medical doctor, Dr. McIntosh, to consult with him. He directed me to Alexia at the crisis pregnancy center. Alexia counseled me, and we read Exodus 4:11, such a vital scripture during this time for me. However, I had a question Alexia wanted Dr. Jackson to answer, so she called him to see if he would see me. I asked him why one of the OB doctors called the baby a "mass" and that the "mass" needed to be removed as soon as possible. The doctor never used the word *abortion*.

Ms. Becky was in a great deal of distress because her obstetrician had recommended an early abortion to avoid the emotional trauma this severely handicapped child could cause her and her family. After all, the child would certainly die immediately after birth. This lady was a sincere Christian woman who did not accept abortion as a solution to ethical dilemmas, but she was severely conflicted by her circumstance. Through her tears she cried out to me asking, "What should I do?"

Again, what would be the compassionate, caring advice to her? Once again, I gave my best advice. I gently and carefully replied, "This unborn child is a baby, a human being created in God's image, with a purpose to glorify God. How you respond to this circumstance is a part of your life testimony and a part of how you glorify God–or not. Your baby's condition is no surprise to God. To paraphrase Psalm 139, 'God created your child's inmost being; He knit your baby together in his mother's womb. We praise God because your baby is fearfully and wonderfully made. God's works are wonderful, and we know that full well. Your baby's frame was not hidden from God when he was made in the secret place. When he was woven together in the depths of the earth, God's eyes saw that baby's unformed body. All of his days are ordained for him and are written in God's book before one of them came to be.'

This is an opportunity for you to make a statement about the value of human life before an audience of medical personnel who may not value life at all. My recommendation is that you deliver your baby and love him in the name of Jesus until he breathes his last breath. It may not be the easy choice, but it will be the right choice. No one

> *My recommendation is that you deliver your baby and love him in the name of Jesus until he breathes his last breath.*

will fault you for choosing an abortion, but you will have to live with your conscience before God for the rest of your life."

She wept giant tears in my office that day and said, "Thank you, Dr. Jackson. I knew that was what I should do. I just needed to hear someone say it." God gave her great grace, and despite the consternation of her OB physician, she carried that baby to term.

BECKY

With the love and help from my Christian friends and a sister in Christ, Catanna Martin, who stood by my side every moment, I delved into God's Word. It is so easy and convenient to let emotions and feelings sway the outcome of decisions. However, the Lord is sovereign and His Word must be obeyed. I knew this truth, so this spiritual battle had to be fought with God's Word and His armor.

Every day I quoted I Corinthians 10:13, which says, "No temptation has overtaken you but such as is common to man; and God is faithful, who will not allow you to be tempted beyond what you are able, but with the temptation will provide the way of escape also, that you may be able to endure it." God was and still is faithful and provided a way to stand and to bear the times when I thought I wouldn't be able to endure.

The Lord's grace was sufficient because His power was strong and perfect in my weakness; therefore, I could boast in the Lord and all He did. My sister in Christ told me the Lord "is doing a new thing," and He "is making a way in the desert," (Isaiah 43:19 NIV). The Lord certainly opened both our eyes, and we learned so much about Him.

Ms. Becky eventually delivered a Trisomy 18 baby who only lived a few hours. She rocked that precious child until he went to be with Jesus. She valued life. All the days (minutes) ordained for her child were written in God's book before one of them came to be. She kept her testimony intact, and she glorified God with her life.

BECKY

Many people told me just to have great faith and all would be okay. Many quoted Romans 8:28; many told me that after the delivery, I could just go back to my normal life. What these people didn't realize was that after the delivery and the years since then, I developed a "new normal" of life, which included compassion for children with disabilities and their parents. I developed a stronger, more mature faith that only the Lord of lords could develop in a person when "praise demands a sacrifice," and a concern for women who aren't grounded in God's Word and who need Christian guidance. Romans 8:28 ("God causes all things to work together for good to those who love God, to those who are called according to His purpose") ultimately came to fruition, but it took a while as healing occurred. Thank God for Christian doctors and Christian crisis pregnancy centers, both of which started me on this ministry trajectory.

She grieved hard for a year and a half before she could speak about this publicly. Eventually, she was able to share her testimony about this situation in church and at the CPC banquet in Spartanburg, at which she shared the emotional difficulty of her decision. Nevertheless, she had no regret regarding giving life to her unborn child, even though only for a few moments of time. What if she had followed the doctor's advice? She would have been just one more Christian with a tainted testimony with no credibility in the eyes of the world, claiming that the unborn child has infinite worth yet discarding her own child when she found out he had a serious defect. She would have been unable to bring any glory to God in this trial, carrying a load of remorse and guilt all of her days because she had worshiped at the altar of moral relativism.

In Deuteronomy 30:19, Moses challenged the people of Israel to "choose life in order that you may live, you and your descendants." Once again, the *the right choice is not always an easy choice, but in the long run it is always the best choice; it brings the blessing of God.*

right choice is not always an easy choice, but in the long run it is always the best choice; it brings the blessing of God.

BECKY

At night after everyone was in bed, I rocked my baby boy while he was still safe in my womb. I prayed that the Lord would be merciful and would not let my son suffer. When I couldn't pray, I quoted Romans 8:26-27. The Lord answered my prayer on the delivery day. He sent a Christian nurse to be with me all day. When my son was born, he never cried but our precious nurse did. When my friend, Catanna (who stayed with me during delivery), handed me the baby to hold, she told me all this confirmed to her that "abortion is not the answer; it is not the right choice."

I unwrapped the blanket and saw my precious baby boy, 4 pounds, 3 ounces with ten fingers and ten toes. My father and stepmother bought the baby a blue outfit to be buried in; at the funeral the gospel was presented. "Jesus Loves Me" and "My Tribute, How Can I Say Thanks" were sung. John 14:6, a special verse to me, was read because it is not only essential for eternal life but also essential for an abundant life while on this earth.

When I go to my son's grave, I see a marker with Jesus holding the children, and I know my son is not in that grave, but is whole and healed in heaven with his heavenly Father. II Corinthians 1:3-5 (NIV) are verses I want to exemplify–"Praise be to the God and Father of our Lord Jesus Christ, the Father of compassion and the God of all comfort, who comforts us in all our troubles, so that we can comfort those in any trouble with the comfort we ourselves have received from God. For just as the sufferings of Christ flow over into our lives, so also through Christ our comfort overflows." To God be the glory!

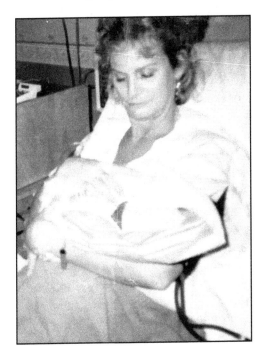

Becky with her baby

Chapter Four

Every Family Should Have One

It snowed in Spartanburg that day—a rare and joyous occasion for us southerners. Standing on the fifth floor of Spartanburg Regional Medical Center at about 8:00 a.m., I looked out over our hometown and watched the white stuff blanket the city. The day had the potential for being especially happy for us, as my wife and I were about to deliver our ninth child. I know what you are thinking, and, no, I did not miss that class in medical school, and, yes, we do know where babies come from!

We chose to have an early ultrasound at fourteen weeks, not because we wanted to know the sex of the baby (the ultrasound was too early anyway, and with nine children we like surprises), but because we hoped to assure our parents that all was well. The ultrasound revealed a normal baby, which we shared with our relieved parents. However, we soon discovered that such ultrasounds are not always correct.

About 10:00 a.m. the fetal monitor began to indicate fetal distress as occasional decelerations of the baby's heart rate occurred. I had planned to deliver the baby since I delivered all but one of our children, but I decided to call in an obstetrician to be on standby just in case we needed an emergency c-section. It seemed the baby wanted to hang up at about six centimeters. We realized the baby was not in the right position, but with my wife lying on her left side to decrease these decelerations, he thankfully moved into position. Our fourth son and ninth child arrived soon into God's world, albeit with the umbilical cord wrapped around his neck twice. I cut the cord to assist with delivery; however, I did not think his oxygen levels had been compromised because the cord was not too tight around his neck.

Upon delivery I handed him to the NICU nurses because he was not breathing on his own and had to be resuscitated with assisted breathing and oxygen for a short period. They assessed his Apgars at two and seven — not so good! They are supposed to be eight and ten in healthy babies! I finished caring for my wife and hurried quickly to the NICU along with everyone else, mainly to check out his breathing. Then I returned to my wife and told her that we had a strong, healthy boy.

After making a few phone calls to tell our family he had arrived, I returned to the NICU where the neonatologists and I examined the baby more closely, and where we began to suspect that my newest Jackson boy was a Downs baby with a loud heart murmur. Nevertheless, he was the cutest little Downs baby anyone had ever seen (in my humble but expert opinion).

My mind drifted back to an experience many years before when I was a resident at that same hospital. I had delivered a handicapped baby to a family with multiple children. Later, I stood at the nursery window with the parents to observe their newborn baby. The mother wept silently as she contemplated the implications of raising a handicapped child with a house full of other children. Her husband stood beside her with his strong arms around her shoulders. He, too, was looking at their obviously abnormal little boy child. Then with a very compassionate voice he said, "Mama, this one is going to need a lot more love." Those words pierced my heart and sank into my mind so that almost twenty years later they returned as I stood looking at my own Downs boy. I suddenly began to smile as God filled me up with love for this precious little boy of mine. Yes, he was going to need a lot more love than all the rest and God would supply it.

I returned to my wife again. She asked me if I was concerned, and I said, "...a little." She knew immediately that I suspected Downs Syndrome, and I watched as my sweet and normally strong, stable wife lost control of her emotions. All I could do at this point was to take us to Jesus. I did the only thing I knew to do, and that was to claim His grace and His sufficiency for all of us. We were going to need it.

CARLOTTA

As soon as my husband, Robert, delivered this last little Jackson munchkin, he held him up for me to see before giving him to the nurse. Normally, I would have been given the baby, but he thought it best to pass him to the nurse this time. After all, he wasn't breathing! When I saw his face, it was clear to me that something wasn't right with this one. His head was swollen and bluish-red, but most obvious were his, oops, oriental-looking eyes. Though neither I nor my husband is Asian, several of our children have had oriental-looking eyes, but these, I told myself, were a little too much so. My mind raced unhappily to the diagnosis of Downs Syndrome. I mean, after all I was forty-four years of age; I shouldn't be surprised, right?

So they carried the baby quickly to the NICU, and soon I was in the delivery room all by myself. What began as a snowy, bright wintry day became a gloomy, dark hospital room for me. I struggled with an angry rejection of my son, my husband, and my God. I struggled because I had already done this. I had been here one time. I had already had one special child. Our marriage, our family had already endured and learned to trust God in the middle of just such a storm. I knew the fears. I knew the responsibilities. I knew what was coming.

In that moment, I did not want to do it again. I'm not going to lie. There have been many such fearful and heavy moments since, but this was the worst one. I did not want yet another handicapped child. Few families in my circle had one special child, and I knew of no one with two! No, God, please, no!

As I write these words seventeen years later, my head sinks into my hands and my tears flow yet again. That little boy is in another room right now–enjoying life, eating his sandwich that he prepared, and talking to himself. I wouldn't trade him for any normal child! He is our treasure.

I wouldn't trade him for any normal child! He is our treasure.

However, I couldn't see the future right then in that dark delivery room. All I could see was a dreadful, bleak sinkhole, so I foolishly descended into an abyss of self-pity and despair, not wanting to believe what had just happened. I wallowed in my humanity there for a while before I realized that I had not fallen into the abyss all alone. In the overwhelming darkness, I sensed the very palpable presence of a loving and compassionate Heavenly Father. Psalm 139 says I cannot escape His presence, even in Sheol. That's where I definitely thought I was, and He was indeed there, just as He promised.

No Bible was within reach of my body, half paralyzed from an epidural, but the verses in my memory rushed to flood my soul with the peace that certainly "surpasses all comprehension," (Philippians 4:6-7). In that moment, He reminded me that He would "never desert [me], nor will [He] ever forsake [me]," (Hebrews 13:5). He reminded me that "my flesh and my heart may fail, but God is the strength of my heart and my portion forever," (Psalm 73:25-26). He reminded me that "...the eyes of the Lord move to and fro throughout the earth that He may strongly support those whose heart is completely His," (2 Chronicles 16:9).

Slowly, I began to climb my way out and to peak out over the edges of life and of my emotional pit to see a loving husband and a tiny, precious baby boy who needed his mommy. Most of all, I saw an enabling God who empowers and sustains. I held onto Him for all I was worth — well, I really should say He held onto me while He brought me under the shadow of His wings with His shepherd's staff and into the cleft of the Rock. Once again, I experienced the fullness of God's grace.

I don't remember if we had chosen a complete name for our new son before he was born or not, but soon we announced to the world that Thomas Jonathan Lee Jackson entered God's world on January 22, 2000, the infamous anniversary of the Supreme Court decision called *Roe v. Wade* legalizing abortion in the United States. Mr. Prolife himself had a Downs baby on this anniversary! Doesn't God have a sense of humor? That's a serious name for a special little boy. Thomas and Lee are family names, but Thomas Jonathan and Lee are also the names of two famous, godly Civil War generals, Thomas Jonathan Jackson and Robert E. Lee. We like to think of Thomas as having a wall in his heart that is like his namesake, "Stonewall" Jackson.

Because he struggled to maintain a normal oxygen level, a doctor ordered an echocardiogram. Robert and I both attended the echo, which revealed a cardiac defect called an A-V canal (essentially no central wall separating the right and left sides of the heart), a common defect for babies with Downs Syndrome. We learned very quickly that Thomas needed a new wall in his heart with this defect, so the goal was to help him gain as much weight as possible in order to help him endure open heart surgery more successfully.

We left the hospital after two days, without our newborn baby for the first time. Thomas came home three days later, sucking ever so slowly from a bottle. I opted not to nurse him as it was more work for him, and he needed the extra calories from boosted formula. The doctors told us to line up donors for eight pints of blood for the eventual surgery, and they put him on Lasix, Lanoxin, and Aldactone for heart failure.

Thus began a ten-week emotional rollercoaster of hospitalizations, cardiologist visits, and several emergency trips in ambulances due to Thomas' persistent congestive heart failure. All the while, we tried to maintain some sense of normalcy for our other eight children. To this day we are thankful for all of the friends who helped us keep life as normal as possible for our children with food, cleaning, ironing, and transportation. You name it–our friends did it.

Thomas struggled to maintain his weight due, in part, to an intestinal blockage called pyloric stenosis for which he had surgery at ten days of age. Then he was diagnosed with severe reflux; plus, he ran the gamut of extremely high temperatures, diarrhea, and vomiting. Every time he ran a fever, the physicians did a sepsis workup, including a spinal tap and antibiotics. Each time, after a few days, he came home looking fairly stable.

One Wednesday night in March, Thomas began to run a fever. However, when I left the next morning, I thought Thomas looked pretty good and the fever had resolved. I felt comfortable going to work. After I left, my wife called to say he had had the worst diarrhea she had ever seen. That was saying something, considering this was our ninth child and we had experienced many episodes of diarrhea over our parenting years. She said it looked like full bottles of undigested formula going straight through him.

My wife had planned to take our other children on a field trip to WLFJ, our local Christian radio station, forty-five minutes down the road, so she set off in that direction. By the time she reached the station, Thomas began to run a temperature and started to look dehydrated. She drove straight to my office as quickly as possible. By the time she got there, he was lethargic and cyanotic. We took him immediately to the hospital, where they began to work on him feverishly, thinking he might not make it. In a few hours he was transferred by ambulance to another city's PICU.

Indeed, Thomas experienced hypovolemic shock from the extreme diarrhea. His kidneys temporarily shut down and his blood work (electrolytes, BUN, and creatinine for the medically inclined) was so off, even the doctors appeared shocked. Then the scariest problem occurred—DIC, disseminated intravascular coagulation, an ominous event. Normal platelet levels are above 150,000. His dropped to a low of 21,000. Thomas began to show blood in his stool and urine, as patients with DIC may spontaneously bleed from every orifice when platelets drop below 50,000. He received a platelet transfusion. This was the third blood component transfusion he had received during his multiple hospitalizations.

Interestingly, my wife, a coronary care nurse twenty-plus years before this, noticed what looked like a serious heart arrythmia cross the heart monitor. She did not know whether to be alarmed or not, considering we can all throw PVCs on occasion, but because of his heart situation, she thought she should report it, which she did. They disbelieved her, but then a nurse saw it happen as well. Stat potassium and digoxin levels were ordered. The dig level was extremely high, which could have accounted for his lethargy and unwillingness to feed. They held his Lanoxin, did an EKG, and put a Holter monitor on him. Everyone around us began to take on increasing tones of concern in their voices for Thomas, for us, for my wife.

The Family Doctor Speaks: The Truth About Life

CARLOTTA

I don't like rollercoasters at amusement parks, but in order to be a "good" mom, I will ride them–with my eyes closed. I certainly did not like the rollercoaster I was on the first weeks of Thomas's life because it was going downhill most of the time. I found myself wishing I could just close my eyes to it all. I also realized how faithless I could be, but in the middle of that revealing discovery, I also remembered how faithful my God is. God's Word is so precious, and just at the right time He took me to 2 Timothy 2:13, which is what I call my "take away" verse from these difficult days. The verse says, "If we are faithless, He remains faithful; for He cannot deny Himself." I may have been faithless, but He was not. He gave me His abiding presence and all of the resources I needed to take care of Thomas. A calm assurance enveloped me much of the time. It was not of me but of God. Practically speaking, I had to rest in the Lord, focus on priorities and forget the rest until the rollercoaster slowed to its final stop.

Miraculously, Thomas stabilized somewhat, recovering from the DIC, but now we knew heart surgery was imminent. He remained in the hospital where one of us had to stay with him at all times. To those friends and family who spent the night in his room to relieve us, we still remember. To those who prayed, we still remember. To those who still ask about Thomas, we treasure your asking. We will never forget. (It's been seventeen years, and I still have patients who prayed for him so long ago who ask how he is doing.)

Thomas's underlying cardiac condition caused a constant mixing of the oxygenated and deoxygenated blood, obviously not normal and not a good thing. This defect required a surgical repair at ten weeks of age at Carolina Medical Center in Charlotte, North Carolina. His surgeon was Dr. Watts of the Sanger Clinic, who provided excellent surgical care. Our family will be forever grateful for Dr. Watts' compassion and surgical expertise.

Within hours of surgery, our previously blue baby became pink and began to feed vigorously. He was able to keep his formula down consistently for the first time in ten weeks. He began to gain weight within days and hasn't stopped gaining for all these years. He came home within a week on oxygen but really didn't need it; however, he did require a feeding tube for sixteen months secondary to reflux.

When Thomas was two years old, he graduated from most of his doctor visits. He became relatively strong and robust, walking at eighteen months although he continued to attend physical, occupational, and speech therapy. He was (and still is) a delightful child who brought smiles and laughter into our home, and we could not get enough of squeezing and hugging that precious little boy.

One day, our then sixteen-year old daughter Rebecca was playing with Thomas on our sofa. She was tickling his ribs just to hear him laugh, a most contagious laugh. Suddenly, she popped her head over the couch and said to my wife and me, "Every family should have a Downs baby."

"Every family should have a Downs baby."

Then she commenced to tickle her youngest sibling once again. My wife and I looked at each other in amazement, wondering how in the world she could say such a thing at such a young age. Would we really wish a Downs baby on every family? We looked at each other and smiled. Yes — a resounding yes! Thomas was, and still is, a great blessing and a great joy to our family even though his first year of life was quite arduous for all of us.

As the years passed, we began to call Thomas "the Professor" because of the lessons learned at his feet, lessons that we probably would not have learned in any other way other than *we began to call Thomas "the Professor" because of the lessons learned at his feet,* having had a Downs child in our family. The professor really has instructed us well. In fact, we often say Thomas is highly intelligent; he came NOT to learn, but to teach.

My children learned to give, expecting nothing in return. Thomas required a great deal of nurturing and a great deal of serving in order to care for his most basic needs. They remember well holding Thomas's feeding bag until their arms grew weary before it emptied. They remember well either traveling with Mom or waiting for her to drive to and from therapies and doctor visits, and all the while babysitting their other siblings. They remember well changing the diaper of an eight-year-old boy. There was no quid pro quo from Thomas, giving something in return, except that he did give the very best hugs.

Our whole family learned to have a servant's heart when dealing with Thomas, something that a lot of my adult friends have not yet learned to acquire. Jesus said He "...did not come to be served, but to serve, and to give His life a ransom for many," (Matthew 20:28). One of the highest virtues of the Christian life is the acquisition of a servant's heart. Thomas, our professor, has taught all of us well the finer points of serving one another.

When our family sees another Downs child, we want to run up to him and hug him and the parents. Our hearts swell with compassion, affection, and understanding. We have an immediate connection with any family that has a handicapped child. We feel compelled to speak to them and share our common experiences. It's almost like the Downs community is one big family with a shared common denominator–our Downs family members.

Why can a Downs child in a family cause tremendous angst? I respectfully submit that our lower natures reject the notion of having to serve another person for the rest of our lives. Our "normal" children will grow up and fly away, but a handicapped child will live with us forever, and we will be required to serve him for the rest of our days. Now seventeen, we call Thomas the "backwards boy" because he still puts his clothes on backwards. Most of the time he can use the microwave properly, but occasionally we have to purchase a new one because he created a burnt offering inside the old one.

Even now we have what we call "Thomas alerts" because he will suddenly and quietly disappear. Unbeknownst to us, just this past winter he left the house and walked down to the river that surrounds our property. After sounding the alert, we found him sitting beside the water with a towel and sunglasses and wearing a life jacket. Even though we live in the south, the dead of winter can be cold in South Carolina! My wife and I envision ourselves driving down to the river when we are eighty-five to search for Thomas! Lord, help us!

The prospect of continuous servitude is what causes most of us angst when faced with the possibility of adding a special needs child to our families. Nevertheless, what Rebecca said is still true: Every family should have a Downs child. Why? A special needs child teaches us lessons in life that we desperately need to learn, and if it takes a special needs child to teach me to be more like Jesus, then so be it. For that matter, it would be a

> *A special needs child teaches us lessons in life that we desperately need to learn,*

good thing if we sprinkled a few Downs children in the midst of our church fellowships. It would be a healthy thing for our church families to learn how to minister to special needs children and adults. It would make us all more like Jesus. If the thought of this makes your heart hurt, then maybe you aren't serious about being like Jesus!

The sad thing is that with modern prenatal diagnostic testing, Downs children can be detected in utero. Between 67 and 92% of Downs babies are aborted, depending upon the country and the accuracy of records, before they see the light of day, before they touch their mama's face, and before they hear their daddy's laughter.[1] Where have all the special needs instructors gone? Where are all the Professor Thomases of this world? Where are the handicapped teachers? They are aborted before they have the chance to teach their first lesson. They are aborted before they minister to us in our churches. They are aborted before we benefit from sitting at their feet. We abort them before God's eternal plan for their lives even begins to be worked out.

What is the measure of a culture? Do we measure a culture by how we treat those who are wealthy or famous or powerful, or do we measure a culture by how we treat those who are the weakest and infirm and powerless? Sorry, but God doesn't use many mighty, wealthy, or wise.

> For consider your calling, brethren, that there were not many wise according to the flesh, not many mighty, not many noble; but God has chosen the foolish things of the world to shame the wise, and God has chosen the weak things of the world to shame the things which are strong, and the base things of the world and the despised, God has chosen, the things that are not, that He might nullify the things

that are, that no man should boast before God.
(I Corinthians 1:26-29)

God chose Gideon to be a judge/leader in Israel. He ultimately led 300 men to a stunning military victory over 20,000 Midianites. What is so surprising is that Gideon was the youngest son in his family, and his family was of the tribe of Benjamin, considered the least significant of the tribes of Israel. Usually, the eldest son would be chosen for a noble task, not the youngest.

Why would God choose the youngest son from the least family in the most insignificant tribe in Israel to accomplish such a great and mighty military victory? It is because He doesn't often choose the mighty, the wealthy, or noble. He delights to use the weak, the foolish, and the despised things of this world to accomplish His eternal purposes. Why? It is because God got the glory, not Gideon. Everyone knew that God had accomplished a mighty military victory, not Gideon. He was a know-nothing farmer.

CARLOTTA

At the time of this writing, we have just celebrated Christmas–a time when we give gifts to one another. On Robert's side of the family we pick names, so family members often pick someone they rarely see and hardly know, making it a little difficult to buy gifts. Never in all of our years of exchanging gifts have I ever heard anyone say, "Take this back; I don't want it. Take this back; I don't need it. Take this back; it's ugly or broken. It's not my cup of tea, or I already have some, thank you very much." If we thought these things, we wouldn't say them. It's just not the polite or right thing to do. But when God, the great Gift Giver, who knows us intimately and knows exactly what we need, starts giving out gifts, which is what Psalm 127 says children are, we have the audacity to say, "Take it back. I don't need him. I don't want her. Children are not my thing. This one is ugly and deformed. I already have some, thank you very much."

To reject or to despise the gift of a child is to despise or reject the Giver. To reject the gift is to reject what God can do through the gift. The gift is a grace gift, and by that I mean the gift works in us the characteristics of grace that we all so desperately need in order to reflect the image of God, the nature of God, and in order to minister to one another and to the lost world. We are the clay, and He is the Potter. He uses the pressures of this life to mold us as He sees fit. He uses children to mold us. (I guess we needed a lot of molding since He gave us nine!)

Thomas (and John Richard) is a special grace gift. This grace gift was given for His glory. IT wasn't because we sinned or Thomas that he has Downs. As Robert said–God often chooses to get glory through the weak and the foolish. May He be glorified in how we all respond to those who are weak and foolish. May He be glorified in a young man named Thomas who lives to serve Jesus in the best way he can and possibly better and purer than the rest of us.

When Thomas was about one and a half years old, I was lying on my bed tossing him up into the air. We were having a BLA, a big loving attack. One of my favorite movies *Chariots of Fire* came to my mind. The grand and glorious music started going through my mind, and I could see Eric Liddel running down the beach speeding up as he ran, then all of a sudden throwing his head back and thrusting ahead of everyone else. Do you remember what he said? About the time he would throw his head back, his words "When I run, I feel His pleasure" would play in the background. Yes, yes, yes! When I threw Thomas up into the air that day, I felt His pleasure. When I changed the diaper of a nine- year old boy, I felt His pleasure. When you lovingly turn a disabled parent, spoon feed your twenty-year old paralyzed daughter, say no to a cocaine addicted son, accept a crisis pregnancy, trustingly learn the diagnosis of a terminal disease, or say goodbye to a loved one, you, too, should feel His pleasure. AND the world is watching–watching to see if your Christian faith makes a difference in how you respond to this fallen world.

When God uses your handicapped child to accomplish His purposes, who gets the glory? Of course, God will. Everyone will know that God did it and will stand back in amazement. More than that, your special needs child will not reach out and touch God's glory and claim it for himself, as you and I are inclined to do. That's why God delights to use the humble, handicapped people among us at times. That's why I pray for my two special boys every day that their lives will be lived "to the praise of the glory of His name."

What about the hard cases? You mean the handicapped children of this world? They just need a little more love– that's all. Oh, and yes, I do agree with Becca. Every family needs a Downs baby. Don't you agree?

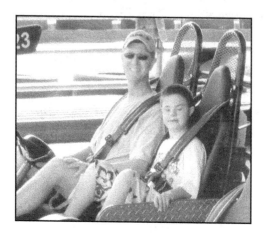

Thomas enjoying life with his dad

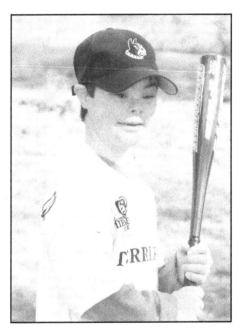

Thomas playing Carolina Miracle League
baseball

Chapter Five

Crossing Over

Wanda was my patient who attended a local church near my office. Her husband was an emergency responder part time and worked at a textile mill full time. They became pregnant after their first two children were already in high school. I was the one who informed her that her pregnancy test was positive. Without hesitation, she informed me emphatically she was not going to have this baby. Without hesitation, I informed her she could not have an abortion without violating her Christian convictions. With fire in her eyes, she told me to mind my own business; it was her own body, and she could do with it as she pleased.

I told her the baby she carried was not her body, but was a separate and unique unborn child created in the image of God. More than that, I told her if she had an abortion the spirit of God would give her a lifetime of remorse and regret. Her response was, "We'll see about that." The next time I saw her, she was no longer pregnant.

Wanda was a Christian woman, a child of the light, who supposedly walked in the light but who crossed over into the darkness. I was deeply saddened by her choice. She continues to see me as a patient, and we have never discussed her decision again.

She has constant problems in her family. I've had to provide frequent marriage counseling for her and her husband because their marriage and their family stay in perpetual turmoil. Their son stays in trouble with the law. Their daughter was pregnant before marriage. Wanda is a loud and brash woman who has hardened her heart towards God and towards biblical truth. I'm afraid that crossing over for her created a lifetime of heartache and sorrow. I don't mean to imply that all of this turmoil is due to a single poor choice involving an abortion. Her life is tumultuous due to many other poor decisions in her life as well. The abortion was just one of many.

I was standing with my family in front of the capitol steps in Columbia, South Carolina, on a blustery, cold January day. It was not the first time we had stood there. In fact, we often go in January to stand in the cold and sometimes in the rain to participate in the annual Right-to-Life March held every year prior to January 22, the anniversary of *Roe v. Wade*. As we stood there on this particular Saturday, we heard a very animated young woman standing on the capitol steps sharing her story. Her name was Abby Johnson.

Ms. Johnson worked at the Planned Parenthood abortion clinic in Bryan, Texas, for eight years, ultimately becoming its director because she had a real desire "to help women in need."[1] She was increasingly troubled, however, as she began to see Planned Parenthood was not so much about helping women as it was about making money.[2] This truth eventually hit home one momentous day and changed her world.

On September 26, 2009, one of the abortion doctors required assistance with an abortion procedure.[3] Finding no one, a coworker asked Abby to help. It just so happened the doctor was performing an ultrasound-guided abortion. Before her horrified eyes, she watched a perfectly formed unborn child visible on the ultrasound screen being suctioned out of the mother's womb and into a glass jar. The visual and audible imagery of that procedure left her completely devastated. She realized in an instant that all of the Planned Parenthood drivel she had been feeding to patients for years had been utterly and completely false.[4]

Ms. Johnson went to her office, shut the door, and pondered the reality that she had "just participated in a death... not a medical procedure."[5] A week passed painfully, sleeplessly, and awkwardly as she went over and over in her mind the ugliness she had seen until she knew she needed help. She headed toward the back door of the Coalition for Life office and called their phone number. She said, "This is Abby Johnson from Planned Parenthood." She paused.

The lady on the other end said, "Well, hi, Abby. I know who you are."

When Abby walked, weeping, through the back door of the crisis pregnancy center, she encountered two shocked CPC workers. She blurted, "I want out. I just can't do this anymore." Abby spent half a day talking to these counselors, pouring out her heart to them and having them pray over her. She never went back to the abortion clinic except to move out.[6] In fact, she is now a much sought after prolife advocate and speaker, and also the founder of And Then There Were None, a ministry to other abortion clinic workers who want out.[7] Yes, Abby Johnson crossed over to the other side.

Ms. Johnson is not the only person who has crossed over. A fellow prolife advocate called me one night and asked me if I would like to eat supper with him. He had some people he would like for me to meet. My wife and I met him at a local restaurant where he introduced me to Flip Benham, who at the time was the director of Operation Rescue, and a delightful lady by the name of Norma McCorvey. Most people would not recognize that name, but she is the Roe in *Roe v. Wade*.

Ms. McCorvey was pregnant out of wedlock in 1970 when the prochoice community was looking for a test case to present to the Supreme Court to hopefully overturn the restrictions on abortion in our country. The young Norma was willing to lend her situation to the National Organization of Women in hopes of obtaining an abortion in the state of Texas, where abortion on demand was not available. Her legal counsel persuaded her to claim she had conceived as a result of rape, which was entirely untrue; nevertheless, that was her story, which lent emotional pathos to her court case.[8] The case took over two years to wend its way through the legal channels; therefore, Norma never had an abortion. Because her counselors wanted her to stay pregnant, they did not advise a naive Norma of her option to go to Mexico for an abortion.[9]

She was given the pseudonym Roe to protect her identity. Little did she know that she would become the Roe in the 1973 Roe v. Wade Supreme Court decision overturning the prolife statutes in all fifty

> *Little did she know that she would become the Roe in the 1973 Roe v. Wade Supreme Court decision*

states. Little did she know her legal case would ultimately lead to the deaths of millions of babies in America over the next forty plus years.

Ms. McCorvey eventually became employed by an abortion clinic in the state of Texas. On March 31, 1995, Operation Rescue moved next door to the clinic where she worked. By divine appointment Ms. McCorvey and Flip Benham, who was by then the president of Operation Rescue, began to meet on a regular basis and they struck up a friendship. By this time, it was too late for her. He had been praying for her for many months, and she realized that all the innuendo spoken about him by the press and employees of NOW was entirely untrue. In fact, she really liked Mr. Benham and became fiercely loyal to him.[10]

In July 1995, after experiencing the unconditional love of Christian prolifers, Norma McCorvey herself became a Christian. She crossed over. She was "transferred from the domain of darkness into the kingdom of God's beloved Son," (Colossians 1:13). She became a believer in the Lord Jesus

Christ. Ms. McCorvey confessed and experienced forgiveness "for allowing [her] name to go on that affidavit...for writing a book celebrating [her] advocacy of abortion...for arguing to keep abortion legal...and for actually participating in hundreds of abortions over the years."[11]

Not everyone crosses from darkness into light. Some people, like Wanda, pass from the light into the darkness. When I used to pray at the abortion clinics, it was not uncommon to see automobiles come through the gates of the clinic with bumper stickers proclaiming allegiance to certain churches nearby. This always caused me a great deal of grief, knowing that someone inside had chosen abortion as a solution to a problem pregnancy, knowing that someone inside had rejected her biblical convictions in favor of death as a solution to her moral dilemma, and knowing that someone inside had crossed over from light into darkness.

I strongly recommend Norma's book *Won by Love,* which is a brutally honest insider exposé of the abortion industry and prochoice community. It also clearly details the power of the gospel and Christian love. We may all have friends who are just as prochoice as Norma McCorvey. We must not despair. We must stop shaking our heads and start praying. If God can change the heart of Ms. McCorvey, He can change the heart of our prochoice friends. It took years of prayer and kindness to break down the walls in Norma's hard heart, but "nothing is too difficult" for our God (Jeremiah 32:17).

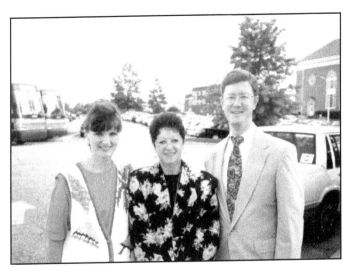

Norma McCorvey and us

Chapter Six

Blind Spots

W e all have blind spots. Blind spots are moral defects in our character we cannot see. Unfortunately, everyone else can see them; we just can't. My wife takes it upon herself to lovingly and persistently point out my blind spots. The problem is ... I can't see them. Sometimes after much prayer and contemplation, the Spirit of God opens my eyes, and I can see myself as God and others see me. Then I am hugely embarrassed, and I say things like, "Was I really like that?"

My children say, "Yes, dad, you really were." Then I want to crawl into a hole forever and never show my face in public again. Now, don't get all puffed up and proud because you have blind spots, too. You just don't see them. That's why they are called blind spots. If you don't believe me, just ask your spouse or your children. They will be glad to fill you in.

What is really sad is when a nation has blind spots–an entire nation. Consider when America's Supreme Court delivered the *Dred Scott v. Sandford* decision in 1857, essentially declaring black people nonpersons or chattel by denying them American citizenship.[1] Looking back from our perspective today, we are incredulous that the Supreme Court justices, all highly intelligent men, could come to such a flawed decision; however, people (even Supreme Court justices) are influenced by cultural and external pressures. No doubt all manner of political, economic, cultural, and racial pressure influenced these justices, but in the end they were blind to the personhood of black people and denied them their rights. Right thinking people today are indignant and appalled at their decision.

Equally appalling was the *Roe v. Wade* decision of January 1973, giving women in America the right to terminate the lives of their unborn children. This decision opened the floodgates to abortion on demand. A former medical partner's wife told me the day after *Roe v. Wade* became the law of the land, every operating suite in the major city hospital where she worked in Chicago was booked for abortion procedures. No routine surgeries occurred for days. The Christian community might have been caught flat-footed, but the prochoice community was ready. The money-grabbing abortion doctors intent on "helping women in need" were ready in an instant to provide abortion services and to open the floodgates.

How could the Supreme Court justices be blind to the personhood of unborn Americans? How could each succeeding generation of Americans be blind to the sacredness and preciousness of the life of little babies in the womb? How could some Americans militantly march in the streets for the right to kill babies under the guise of women's rights? How blind can we be?

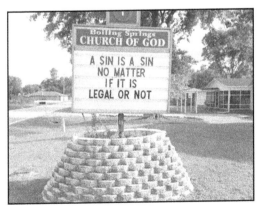

A local church sign that caught my attention

Back in the 1990s, a blind man walked into my office. No, he wasn't physically blind, but he was certainly spiritually blind although he didn't realize it at the time. He had just moved to Spartanburg from Alaska along with a beautiful Asian woman, who accompanied him to my office. As was my habit, I asked, "Where do ya'll go to church?"

He stared at me like a calf looking at a new gate, and answered, "Huh, we don't go to church."

To which I responded, "You mean ya'll don't ever go to church?"

Again he stared at me quizzically and retorted, "Well, no, Doc, I've been an outlaw all my life. I've never even been to church."

After many years of medical practice, I wasn't really surprised, but I continued, "Where did you get married, then?"

He glanced over at his companion and then back to me, and replied, "Well, I've been married five times, but I've never been married in a church."

"What about a wedding chapel?"

He looked at the ceiling for a moment, and then replied, "No, not even in a wedding chapel." It turns out he was not even married to the woman who was with him. Here again was a man like the woman at the well, married five times, divorced five times, and not married to the current woman! So the natural thing for me to do was to invite him to my church. To my astonishment, he agreed to come.

What I did not know then but John revealed to me later was that he was on a spiritual journey at the time. His best friend in Alaska had committed suicide a short time before he left there for South Carolina. While in a motel in Oklahoma, he had watched a one-hour video produced by Focus on the Family describing the life of Harold Morris, who had written a book entitled *Twice Pardoned*. In the video, Morris describes being sent to life in prison in Georgia for being an accomplice to a murder. While in prison, he became a believer in the Lord Jesus Christ. He began a ministry to other inmates that so impressed the governor of Georgia that he was ultimately pardoned. Hence, the title of his book–he was pardoned by the Lord Jesus and by the governor of Georgia.[1]

The Holy Spirit had planted the seed of the gospel in John's heart in the motel room in Oklahoma, unbeknownst to me. Also, a key factor in connecting John, Harold Morris, and me was that I was from a small town in the lower part of the state of South Carolina forty-five miles from Harold Morris' hometown of Beaufort, South Carolina. Almost identical to Harold Morris', my southern drawl attracted John to me. When I began to talk with him about spiritual matters, he was immediately willing to listen. Although I found it odd that this complete stranger from Alaska would be so receptive to a gospel presentation, it later became clear to me that God was orchestrating the movements of all the players in this spiritual drama.

On Sunday he showed up in my Sunday School class where I taught a lesson on Ephesians 2:8-9, which says, "For by grace you have been saved through faith; and that not of yourselves, it is the gift of God; not as a result of works, that no one should boast." At that time my class was a group of young men who did not pay me a lick of attention that particular Sunday morning because they were constantly cutting their eyes over towards the young woman by John's side. However, his attention was zeroed in on my every word.

Later in the worship service, our pastor preached a sermon from II Kings 5 entitled "Seven Ducks in a Muddy River" about Naaman, the Syrian cleansed from leprosy by bathing seven times in the Jordan River. As soon as he finished preaching, John walked straight down the aisle and said, "I want to be a Christian." I was a bit taken aback because as far as I could tell this was his first exposure to the gospel (remember, I did not know yet about his acquaintance with Harold Morris's story). I asked John, "Are you sure? We're talking about giving all of your life to Jesus for the rest of your life."

John was very confident when he said to me, "That is exactly what I want to do." He immediately knelt at the front pew to receive Christ as the Lord of his life.

As time passed, I learned something more about John's previous life. When he was fifteen, he left home never to return, traveling with the carnival for many years. He had been arrested in many states for various offenses and eventually ended up in Reno, Nevada, working in a casino. He was so good at what he did that in a few years time he was a casino manager. Ultimately, he began to manage five casinos and five restaurants. He told me when one is a casino manager in Reno he never pays for food, booze, drugs, or women. He was like a king in Reno for years until he got caught embezzling from a casino. He had to flee for his life in the middle of the night and then went to Alaska, where he opened up an after hours illegal gambling establishment. Gradually, he became quite wealthy there, but he left financially broke when the oil boom collapsed. After his best friend committed suicide, he left to come to Spartanburg, where he met me.

John was radically transformed by his new life in Jesus Christ. For a short while after he became a believer, he continued to work in a small saloon in Spartanburg, dealing cards to make ends meet. On Sundays after church, he ate lunch at my house then left to work in the saloon. I never said anything to John about this, leaving it to the Spirit of God to bring about conviction in his life.

So every Sunday John and his girlfriend ate with my five children, my pregnant wife, and me. So here was the runway model and the king of gambling — who used to parcel out $50–$100,000 in perks to high rolling gamblers to entice them to attend his casinos — sitting down to eat mashed potatoes, fried okra, and meatloaf with a homeschooling family who memorized scripture and worked through the catechism with five children under the age of ten every Sunday lunch. What was he thinking? What a culture shock- for all of us!! What a sense of humor our God has! I bet the angels in heaven were belly laughing every Sunday lunch!

After about six weeks, I noticed John did not leave early after lunch one Sunday. A bit puzzled, I queried, "Aren't you going to be late for your afternoon job?"

He replied, "I don't have that job any longer."

"So what happened to your job?"

"I gave it up; I did not think it was appropriate for a Christian to work in a saloon." That was all either one of us ever said about it.

To our surprise, John also announced he had told his runway model girlfriend that unless she became a believer in Christ, they could not continue their relationship and she would need to return to her home. Filled with consternation, she could not understand him at all; neither could she understand the spiritual concept of being born again. We shared the gospel with her. We prayed with her. We cried with her — all to no avail — at least as far as we ever knew. Ultimately, John bought her a one-way ticket back to her family; and that was all either one of us ever said about it.

Several days later, I invited John to attend a prolife rally in Greenville, South Carolina. We rode with about twelve other people in a little, old church van with holes in its floor. It was freezing cold in January, and the van had no heat; that van needed to go to a church van graveyard. As we rode, John started laughing. I asked, "What are you laughing at?"

He replied, "If my old friends could just see me now!"

I said, "Why?"

In a very serious voice, John replied, "All of my life, I thought abortion was the best thing that could happen to women, and now I find myself riding in a church van with a bunch of Baptists going to a prolife rally." Continuing to laugh, he again said, "If my old friends could see me now!" I pondered his statement for a moment, then I began to laugh as well; and that was all either one of us ever said about it.

What happened to John? I never talked to him about abortion. I never debated with him about the abortion issue. I never even discussed any moral issues with John, up to that point. So what happened? I'll tell you: the Holy Spirit of God illumined his mind, and he was transferred from the domain of darkness into the kingdom of God's beloved Son. He was transferred from darkness into light. John was born again into God's kingdom; now he could see the light and walk in the light. He went from being a prochoice, pro-death advocate who thought that "abortion was the best thing that ever happened to women" to being a prolife advocate in a few days' time, without the benefit of any discussion. First Corinthians 2:14 says, "But a natural man does not accept the things of the Spirit of God; for they are foolishness to him, and he cannot understand them, because they are spiritually appraised."

When I first began to speak in churches, making presentations about the medical and biblical perspective on the prolife issue, I used to take with me a three-foot tall poster depicting a twelve-week gestation infant in the amniotic sac. One day, my three-year old daughter Rebecca saw that poster board before I left to make a presentation in a local church. After she saw the poster, she responded, "Oh, daddy, look at the little baby."

I immediately looked at my wife, and said, "Why can't the doctors, lawyers, judges, and Indian chiefs see what my three-year old daughter can clearly see?" The answer is my little daughter was not hindered by the spiritual blindness affecting the culture at large. She saw what John saw when God opened his eyes. John and Rebecca saw clearly that that which grows in the mother's womb is a baby because their eyes were opened by the Spirit of God. No amount of debate or logic or education will win this issue in the public or political arena. If that were true, the ultrasound machine — that magical window into the womb — would have settled this issue a long time ago.

The ultrasound machine gives amazingly clear pictures of the baby growing in the mother's womb. This machine makes it plain from early on, for all to see, that that which grows in the mother's womb is a baby, a miniature human being. Debate closed. No further discussion.

So why is there further debate? Why are people still adamant about women's rights? Why can't our judges and legislators see what you and I plainly see on these third and fourth generation ultrasound pictures? The answer is because they are spiritually blind. They cannot see the truth. "The natural man does not accept the things of the Spirit of God..." (I Corinthians 2:14).

That is why evangelism is so fundamental to what we as Christians do in every area of our lives. Only when our legislator or judicial friend is born again into the kingdom of God will he see the truth about the sanctity of human life, just like John, without any debate. The Holy Spirit will reveal the truth to them. Just stand back and watch. The same is true for your coworker and your aggravating, know-it-all brother-in-law. Just share Jesus with them in love over time until they are born again. Then watch them come over to your side on a whole host of moral and ethical issues, and watch what happens when God takes the spiritual blinders from their eyes. They will say things like, "I can't believe I used to believe things like that. Did I really think like that? I can't believe I was so blind. If only my old friends could see me now," as they ride in a crippled, old church van on the way to their first prolife rally.

Chapter Seven

Intercession

Understand clearly–the measure of the culture is not what we do with the rich, powerful, or famous, but what we do with the weakest, poorest, and most infirm among us. The challenge for us is to hold up a high standard and to become the champions of the weak, the infirm, and the handicapped. Our challenge is to come alongside of them and to be their voices, their advocates.

Pamela came into my office at sixteen weeks pregnant. Her boyfriend, a heavy beer drinker and a member of a motorcycle gang, browbeat her for several months to obtain an abortion. She was a waitress at a restaurant, barely surviving financially. Her father was a Baptist preacher and, although he was very disappointed in her, he encouraged her to do the right thing, which was to keep the baby. Her father promised to support her financially. He encouraged her to break the ties with her boyfriend whom he considered to be unworthy of her affection. She was too far along to obtain an abortion at the local abortion clinic and realized that to obtain a late-term abortion she would have to go to Atlanta.

I met with Pamela every week for about four weeks for counseling and prayer. I also referred her to the local crisis pregnancy center, where she received additional counseling and prayer. It was evident she wanted an abortion about as much as a bear wanted to put his paw into a bear trap, because she had grown up believing abortion was murder. Yet she desperately wanted to keep her relationship with her boyfriend. She was afraid if she did not abort the baby she would lose him. I shared with her the very real statistic that most unmarried relationships break up after abortions, terrifying her even more.[1]

Despite the counseling and the praying, Pamela broke my heart one Friday afternoon when she notified me of her decision to travel to Atlanta for an abortion on Saturday morning. She and I had become very close during our sessions. We had prayed together and discussed the issue on multiple occasions. I prayed for her repeatedly over the weekend.

To my surprise, she called on Monday to say she was still pregnant. With delight, I asked her what happened. She responded, "I went to the Atlanta abortion clinic, but when I checked in, I had a fever. Upon examination, they found I had a urinary tract infection. They gave me an antibiotic and told me to return in two weeks. While driving back from Atlanta, I prayed and decided to keep my baby." She also decided the boyfriend was not worth the life of her unborn child and she wanted me to deliver the baby. A couple of months later, I delivered her newborn baby girl without any complications and had the privilege of caring for her little girl for a couple of years; then I lost contact with them for a while.

At the same time Pamela pondered the fate of her pregnancy, I shared her situation with my Wednesday night prayer group at my church (anonymously, of course). Now, you have to understand the fifty to seventy folks gathered at Rock Hill Baptist Church in Inman, South Carolina during the 1990s were not your average Wednesday night crowd. Those folks were real prayer warriors. They got on their knees every Wednesday night, took hold of the horns of the altar, prayed for lost people by name, and told God they wouldn't let go until the lost were saved, the sick were healed, and families were restored. During this time we saw numerous answers to prayer, including salvations (my brother, for one) and restored marriages.

For about six weeks we prayed for my patient. I even told her fifty people at my church were praying for her to make the right decision. The women especially prayed, with "groaning too deep for words," on behalf of this mom and for her unborn child. Nevertheless, she felt compelled to go to Atlanta for an abortion. Well, you already know the end of the story. I have no doubt God heard the prayers of fifty-plus prayer warriors, the prayers of the women at the CPC, my prayers, and her father's prayers on behalf of that precious unborn child. Her bladder infection didn't occur by accident. It occurred as a direct result of divine intervention brought on by intercessory prayer! Jesus said, "And all things you ask in prayer, believing, you shall receive," (Matthew 21: 22). Either that is true or it is not. Either we believe that or we don't. The effectiveness of intercessory prayer hangs on the veracity of that statement and the faith of the intercessor. We chose to believe, God intervened, and that little baby survived.

Moses is a biblical hero when it comes to intercession. He constantly fell on his face before God to intervene on behalf of the children of Israel because they had angered God for one reason or another; they complained about the food (manna), they complained about the lack of water in the desert, and even his sister Miriam complained about Moses' spiritual authority. She ended up with leprosy and Moses had to cry out to God on behalf of his sister, i.e., intercession.

We learn a lot from Moses. It didn't bother him to fast for forty days on the top of Mt. Sinai, not once but twice, in order to hear from God on behalf of the people. Also, he persevered in intercessory prayer for a very stubborn and rebellious people on whom God seemed ready to give up. Yet, Moses continued to pray for them, begging God not to give up on His own chosen people. Moses was passionate. In distress and with anger, he tore his clothes and pulled out his beard on multiple occasions as he stood between God and the people, begging God to relent from His anger. It's obvious Moses didn't trifle with sin. He couldn't tolerate the sinful conduct of the people who were called to be the holy representatives of God Himself and who God gave him to lead to the Promised Land.

We derive three important principles of intercessory prayer from the life of Moses: 1) perseverance in prayer, 2) passion in prayer, and 3) purity in prayer. I am convinced God honors the perse-

God honors the persevering, pure-hearted prayer of a passionate prayer warrior

vering, pure-hearted prayer of a passionate prayer warrior who intercedes for the people he or she loves. All three of these elements are essential if we would be intercessors like Moses. Confess your personal sin before the Lord to ensure that you are a pure-hearted prayer warrior and, as Jesus said, "...pray and not to lose heart..." (Luke 18:1). Persevere in prayer on behalf of your family member or friend. I don't necessarily recommend that you tear your clothes or pull out your beard, but God still honors and respects passion in your prayer life.

Many years later when Pamela's daughter was nineteen years old, Pamela brought her to see me for a minor illness. When I walked in the exam room, I saw the daughter dressed in gothic dress; her hair was jet black, she wore the blackest eyeliner, black lipstick, and black fingernail polish. She looked like she had fallen face first into a fishing tackle box because every part of her face was pierced with metal objects, even her tongue. More than this, she had a terrible attitude towards her mother, but *she was alive. She was alive!*

I could tell the mother was extremely proud of her daughter, who was actually quite an attractive young lady despite the gothic attire and metal accoutrements. I really never was quite sure why she actually brought her daughter to my office, because an exam revealed minor symptoms that could have been diagnosed and managed at home. I suspect she wanted to show off her very attractive daughter and to allow me to see the product of all of my praying and counseling!

———————— • ▬ ··◆·· ▬ • ————————

When I began my medical practice, I interviewed a teenage girl who was several months pregnant and unwed. It was obvious to me that she had no intention of pursuing an abortion, so I tentatively asked her what prompted her to maintain the pregnancy even though she was unmarried. She immediately informed me a woman had showed her high school class a prolife film a couple of years previously. She said she was so impressed by the images of unborn children in the womb that she decided right then she would never obtain an abortion. Sadly, she had not made up her mind to preserve her moral purity until marriage.

I found out the woman who showed the film in her school was a fellow right-to-life worker in the local Citizens for Life group that actually met in my office one night per month. This led me to realize we never know the impact of our educational efforts in the lives of other people. Furthermore, we should never cease to educate each succeeding generation of young people about the value of life and the truth about abortion. I later showed this same film in dozens of churches in South and North Carolina.

To say it again, none of us should ever underestimate the power of intercessory prayer and saying the right thing

———— • ▬ ··◆·· ▬ • ————

We should never be afraid to speak the truth about the value of the unborn child

———— • ▬ ··◆·· ▬ • ————

at the right time in a person's life. The Bible says that our speech should always be "seasoned ...with salt," (Colossians 4:6) and that we should always "[speak] the truth in love," (Ephesians 4:15). We should never be afraid to speak the truth about the value of the unborn child and his life.

If we love people without telling them the truth about their situation, we become compromisers. If we tell them the truth without love in our hearts, we come across as condemning. It is a balancing act that none of us gets perfect all the time, but we have to try by God's grace to get it right. Each of us may one day have an opportunity to stand in the gap for the life of an unborn child. We should not draw back. We never know when our intercessory prayers, or speech, seasoned with salt, might be the preservative of the life of an unborn child.

Chapter Eight

Compassionate Christians In Action

"Pastor Fred, why is there no abortion clinic in Spartanburg like the ones in Greenville?"

"Well, actually, there used to be one."

"No kidding. When?"

"About five years ago."

"What happened?"

"Several Protestant pastors and several Catholic men and women picketed every Saturday morning for a couple of months until the property owner decided it was too much bad publicity and he closed it down!"

"No kidding?"

"No kidding."

"Well, I'll be."

I was attending a monthly Spartanburg Citizens for Life meeting held in the waiting room of my medical office in 1986 where I asked the first question of Rev. Fred Thompson. He was a Presbyterian Church of America pastor friend who was active in the prolife movement and was, in fact, one of those Protestant pastors who picketed the abortion clinic in Spartanburg. Those pastors and the Catholic men and women who assisted them are my heroes. Every God-fearing, right-thinking Christian person in Spartanburg County should hold them in the highest regard. Because of their quick, obedient response to God's leading, we don't have a clinic in our county killing thousands of unborn children per year like the one next door in Greenville County. Thank the Lord and thank these Christian activists.

For the record, those prolife heroes were Josephine Barron, Aileen and George Dawson, Carmella Steele, Fred Thompson, and Jack Giddings. Josephine, Aileen, George, and Carmella represented a Catholic church in our community. Both Fred and Jack were PCA pastors. They not only picketed at the abortion clinic, but they engaged the young women in conversation. They offered them options to abortion, even though there was no organized CPC in Spartanburg at that time. They held a baby shower at Roebuck Presbyterian Church and collected baby and maternity clothes and diapers to offer to the young mothers to remove any financial reasons for having an abortion. This was genuine love in action!

Shortly after the above conversation, our Citizens for Life group participated in a nationwide pastors' protest against abortion. We helped to organize the event with a march in our city. Approximately forty pastors attended in order to register our protest against abortion. The local news reported the event. The entire time we were organizing the protest the Holy Spirit was saying to me, "You must provide a viable option to abortion. Merely protesting is not enough." However, I had no idea at the time what that meant.

About this same time, someone gave me a copy of Jerry Falwell and Mel White's book *If I Should Die Before I Wake*. It delineated

Carlotta, I think God is leading me to start a CPC."

the abortion crisis in America but, more importantly, the book described the network of crisis pregnancy centers and maternity homes Liberty Baptist Church, Falwell's church, supported around the country.[1] These centers and homes provided–guess what?–viable options to abortion for young women in unplanned or crisis pregnancies. As I finished the book, I put it down and said to my wife, "Carlotta, I think God is leading me to start a CPC."

She replied, "What is a CPC?"

I responded, "I'm not really sure, but I'm pretty certain that's what God wants me to do." Looking back on it, I laugh at that scene because I had no connections in Spartanburg. I had lived there only five years, four as a resident at the regional hospital and one in private practice. I was not from the upstate of South Carolina; plus, I had no financial resources nor did I know anyone who did. However, I did know the God of the heavens and the earth, and I was willing to be obedient to His leading. Unbeknownst to me, He had been calling a young Wesleyan pastor at the same time He was calling me.

As I confided in the Citizens for Life group at the next monthly meeting my concern for starting a CPC, one of the Catholic women, Joan Cutler, referred me to this pastor named Gene Burgess. Actually, she mentioned him to me in three consecutive meetings, but I didn't pay any attention until the third meeting. This time she took me by the shoulders, shook me like a little dog, and with exasperation she said, "I'm telling you, doctor, call Gene Burgess right now!" Well, I could recognize when the Spirit of the Lord was speaking to me through a dear sister. I left the meeting and called him immediately.

We met at my office the next day where we shared our same burden for ministering to young women in unplanned pregnancies and the same vision for starting a CPC. In fact, he had already begun a 501C3 organization called Hope for Tomorrow's Child with a board of directors, and he had raised $1,400. I could hardly contain my excitement at meeting someone who shared the same vision for ministering to young women in crisis pregnancies. We got on our knees in my office and prayed fervently together that God would make our common vision come true. God forged a true friendship between us that day, lasting now for over thirty years. As "iron sharpens iron," (Proverbs 27:17) so has Gene sharpened my life in many ways.

Gene was way ahead of me because he had a teenager in his church who had conceived a child with his girlfriend. He came to Gene as his pastor for help. Consequently, Gene began to make calls around the county and found few resources available at the time for counseling or financial aid for teenage girls with unplanned pregnancies. Out of curiosity, he put an ad in the paper saying, "Pregnant? Need help?" with his home phone number, and then he promptly forgot about it and left town for the weekend.

His wife, Kathy, totally unaware of the advertisement, received a dozen phone calls from distraught teenage girls requesting help over that weekend while he was away. This was before cell phones, so Kathy had to wait until he returned to town "to let him have it," which she promptly did upon his return. They laugh about it now, but it wasn't funny to his wife then! Nevertheless, he had his answer. Plenty of young women in Spartanburg County needed help with their unplanned pregnancies. God gave him a vision similar to mine. What I find most amazing is God kept bringing other people along who shared the same vision and were way smarter and more talented than Gene or I. God brought board members, directors, volunteers, staff members, and donors. You name it, God provided it. His name is Jehovah Jireh, the Lord who provides.

The first step we had to take after we recruited board members was to raise money for day-to-day operations. We decided to have a fund-raising march with each participant raising pledges from friends and family for each mile they marched. We had ninety-nine participants. On the day of the march we were in high spirits. Not even the morning-long deluge of rain could dampen our spirits nor stop anyone from completing the march, even Lilly Mae Garrett, who was in her seventies and our oldest participant. We raised $10,000. We were in business!

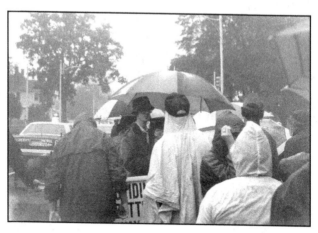

Our first fundraising march

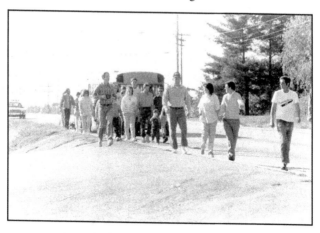

An early fundraising march–in the sun!

Dr. Dick Plummer, a friend of the ministry, donated office space for our first year; we officially opened in February 1987. Sandra Hill was our first director. She told us she had to play the radio when counseling with clients in order to provide confidentiality, since the counseling room was not soundproofed. Hope for Tomorrow's Child was open part time, and we provided services to thirty-four clients our first year.

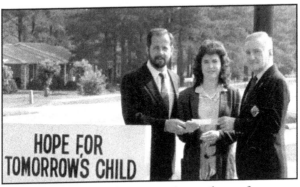

Sandra with Dr. Plummer and a gentleman from
Knights of Columbus

The second year we moved to a larger flat in the Metro Center, where we stayed for a couple of years. Dr. Thornburg (a radiologist and board member), Gene, and I met every Friday morning at 6:00 a.m. in that location to pray for the ministry and for each other. We all grew in the Lord by leaps and bounds due to the accountability we provided for one another. The memory of those early morning prayer meetings is still precious to me. No doubt those prayers also established a strong foundation for the ministry.

Eventually, we graduated from marches to banquets. Six hundred people attended our first banquet with Cal Thomas as our speaker. It was a very nice dress-up affair and well received by our donors. Over the years the banquets grew to be quite large events with between 800-2,000 people in attendance. It became the gala Christian social event of the year in our community. It still is! Imagine that–a prolife fundraising event becoming that popular and that well attended! Isn't God good!

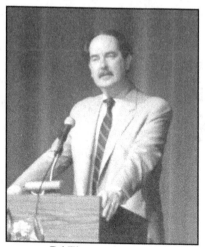

Cal Thomas–our first
banquet speaker

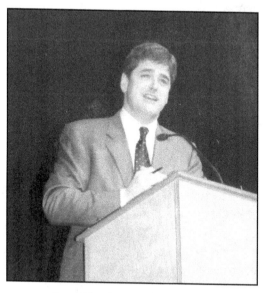

Sean Hannity–another speaker

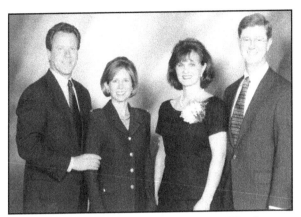

Speaker Governor David and Mary Wood
Beasley with us

For one banquet, I was slated to introduce our speaker for the evening. I dressed up in my black dinner jacket and bow tie, but before I could leave the house, the hospital called to say one of my pregnant patients was in labor and would deliver imminently. "Please hurry!" they exclaimed. I drove quickly to the hospital dressed up like a mannequin, and ran up five flights of stairs and into the delivery room.

"Dr. Jackson, you better hurry. Your patient is crowning. She is going to deliver this baby in a minute. No time to change clothes. Put on these sterile gloves and get in there," exhorted the charge nurse as she hustled me along.

With no time to scrub or put on a surgical gown, I slipped on the sterile gloves and stood in position to assist in the delivery. Sure enough, the baby's head was presenting and with two good pushes the mom delivered a beautiful baby girl into my waiting hands. Now, every obstetrician knows that after the newborn is delivered there is often a gush of amniotic fluid that follows. Knowing this to be true and realizing I had no surgical gown to protect my jet black shoes and pants, I positioned myself as far to the left as I could, and like a skilled matador I lifted my right foot up behind me as high as I could to avoid the gush of fluid as I deftly laid the baby on the mother's abdomen. I caught the eye of the surgical tech, who was grinning from ear to ear behind her surgical mask. Her response—"Ole, well done, doctor!"

The mother arose from her medication-induced fugue state, spied me in my dinner jacket, and sleepily commented, "Dr. Jackson, you look so pretty. Do you dress up like this for all of your deliveries?"

"No, ma'am. Just for my special patients like you."

Before she fell back asleep, she said, "Ohhhh, that's so nice."

Because I am a family doctor, I was also the baby's doctor, so I then examined the baby to ascertain her health, as well as to assure myself the mother was well. After writing orders for both mom and baby, I dashed off to the CPC banquet. I walked into the auditorium as Alexia, our director, called my name while she desperately looked around the audience for me, the one designated to introduce the speaker for the night. I entered the door, calmly walked to the podium, introduced the speaker, and sat down to eat my cold, rubber chicken. No one except my wife and the OB nurses was any the wiser! Yes, God is good and He has a sense of humor!

What was the compelling force behind the founding of our crisis pregnancy center? Heartbreak—for one. We studied the demographic abortion statistics before we launched the ministry, which by this time had become Carolina Pregnancy Center. In 1986, the year Gene and I met, data from the Centers for Disease Control and state health departments reported 12,174 in-state abortions and 49,604 live births in South Carolina, which is a 19.7% abortion rate.[2] These numbers broke our hearts. We knew that God was looking over the ramparts of heaven with tears in His eyes and a grieving heart to see that almost 20% of all pregnancies in South Carolina were ending in abortion.

The number of abortions peaked at 14,133 in-state abortions in 1988 with 53,285 live births, a 23.6% abortion rate.[3]

Just as disturbing were the out-of-wedlock births. The earliest statistics available to me at this time revealed a total of 19,335 live births to unmarried mothers in 1993, a peak of 29,797 in 2008, and 26,741 in 2013 in South Carolina.[4] According to this same DHEC chart, this represents 47.1% of all live births.[5]

We were also motivated by compassion for all of the moms who had come to us after their abortions and said to us, "Why didn't someone tell me it would be like this?" as they shared their remorse and regret for having aborted their babies. Indeed, the emotional pain of abortion is well documented, with one anecdotal story after another in a book I recently read, *Forbidden Grief: The Unspoken Pain of Abortion.* The stories moved me to tears once again. Writing the foreword to the book, Dr. Laura Schlessinger says, "Abortion is a tragic, traumatic act that leaves lifelong scars on women's lives, some of which are not apparent for quite a long while."[6] Yes, it was our responsibility to speak the truth in love, even if some would not care to listen.

Finally, we were compelled by obedience to the manifest will of God. The Scriptures say, "Rescue those being led away to death; hold back those staggering towards slaughter. If you say, 'But we knew nothing about this,' does not he who weighs the heart perceive it? Does not he who guards your life know it? Will he not repay each person according to what he has done?" (Proverbs 24:11-12 NIV) What else could we do? You might be interested to know that since those early days of the prolife movement in South Carolina, thirty-nine crisis pregnancy centers exist around the state according to today's South Carolina Citizens for Life stats.[7] I was privileged to have a small part in starting four of them.

Prolife legislators in South Carolina have passed multiple pieces of prolife legislation designed to protect women and the unborn, including the most recent called the Pain-Capable Unborn Child Protection Act, which Governor Nikki Haley signed on June 8, 2016.[8] Prolife education has progressed unabated for thirty-plus years in churches and schools. As a result, the demand for abortion services has declined significantly in South Carolina with the latest CDC/state data showing 5,878 in-state abortions in 2013 and 57,159 live births, a 13.6% rate.[9] Only three official abortion clinics remain in Charleston, Columbia, and Greenville.[10]

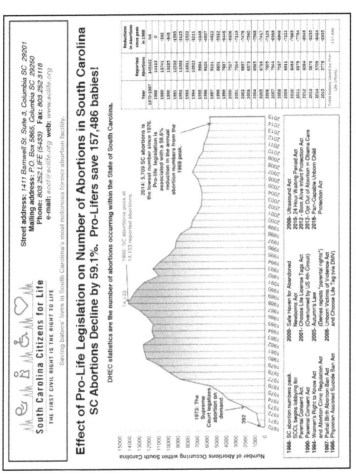

(Used by permission of Holly Gatling, Executive Director,
South Carolina Citizens for Life)

My commitment is to protest abortion until abortion is illegal in America and no child dies by abortion in our country. Do you think that is impossible? Is anything too difficult for God? The black slaves in America thought they would never be emancipated. The children of Israel languished four hundred years in Egypt crying out to God, thinking their cruel bondage would never end. Is God's ear so dull that it cannot hear? Is His arm so short that He cannot save? Oh, ye of little of faith. Pray every day that God will end abortion in America by divine fiat for His glory in such a way that everyone knows there is a God in Israel. May the righteous rejoice and may the wicked be put to shame.

In April 1989, the board of the CPC made our best decision of all time when we hired Alexia Newman to be our director. She has been a godsend to our CPC and our entire prolife community, as well as our community at large. She is a wise, biblically informed, spirit-filled Christian woman who leads our volunteers and staff in prayer, counseling, service, evangelism, and hospitality. In short, she is the bomb!! We love her to the moon and back!

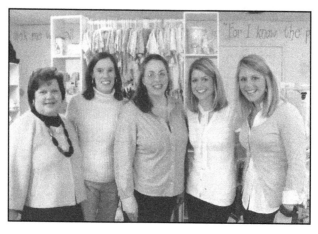

Alexia (far left) with her staff–2008

We moved across the street in the Metro Center to our current location and over time spread out to the entire building, providing crisis pregnancy counseling, post abortion counseling, and "Earn While You Learn" classes that teach young moms parenting skills and provide credits to purchase items from our maternity store. We teach our volunteers all about providing options to young moms in crisis pregnancies and how to delicately share the gospel with them.

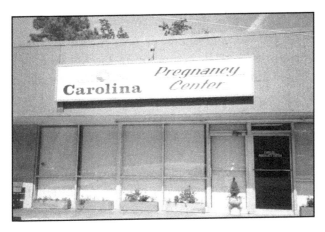

Most recent CPC location

From the beginning we viewed CPC as an extension of the local churches in Spartanburg County, since all of our support comes from churches and individuals. Our mission is to speak the truth in love to women in crisis pregnancies, which inevitably involves sharing the truth about Jesus' ability to transform our lives. Many of our clients will never step off the merry-go-round of immorality and irresponsibility if they are not born again into the kingdom of God, transferred from the domain of darkness into the kingdom of God's beloved Son, and made new creations in Jesus Christ. Otherwise, we'll provide a free pregnancy test, confidential counseling, and they will be back in six to twelve months in another crisis. If there is no change in their hearts, there will be no change in their lifestyles. The heart of the human problem is the problem of the human heart. For "the heart is deceitful...and desperately wicked; who can know it," (Jeremiah 17:9 KJV).

The CPC is a redemptive ministry, and we are committed to speaking the life-changing truth of the gospel of Jesus Christ into the lives of our clients whenever given permission to do so. Every year, approximately ten percent of our 1,200 clients per year confess Christ as Savior due to the evangelistic efforts of our counselors. We do our best to connect them with pastors and churches near where they live who will help them grow in grace and in the knowledge of the Lord Jesus Christ. That is the most exciting part of what the CPC does.

Once again, it is inappropriate to point an accusing finger at young men and women caught in an unplanned pregnancy and simply say, "You shouldn't have an abortion," if we aren't willing to come alongside them with compassion and meaningful, viable options. That is what the CPC is all about–meaningful options provided in a loving way. For many women in an unplanned pregnancy, good options do not exist. Every option has unacceptable consequences, but we should help them take abortion off the table and eliminate it as an option. With our compassion and support, why should anyone perceive killing her/his child as an appropriate option?

You can make a difference in the life of a mother and child. You can be a compassionate Christian activist. Call your local CPC and volunteer to be a counselor, answer the phone, organize the clothes closet, or whatever. Every CPC functions with volunteer efforts. Call them today–before Joan Cutler takes you by the lapels and shakes you like a little dog!

RESOURCES (for finding a CPC)

"Find a Center Near You",
www.sclife.org/#!crisis-pregnancy-centers/csu2

Care Net
44180 Riverside Parkway, Suite 200
Lansdowne, Virginia 20176
Phone: 703.554.8734
Email: info@care-net.org

Lifecall
1.800.noabort or 1.800.662.2678
Text: SHELTER to 313131
Email: mail@lifecall.org

Chapter Nine

Restoration

"Dr. Jackson, can you keep a secret?"
Taken aback by the abrupt question, I responded, "Yes, ma'am, everything you tell me is quite confidential. I'm very good at keeping secrets."

The tall, attractive brunette pondered my statement for long moments, reading my face before she seemed satisfied. With a deep breath and tears forming in her dark brown eyes, she launched into her story. "Every year they ask me at church to teach Sunday School, but I turn them down because I have blood on my hands. Dr. Jackson, I'm a murderer. I killed my own baby. Twenty-five years ago, before I was married, I became pregnant. Out of fear and shame, I obtained an abortion. Nobody knows it. Not my parents. Not my husband. Nobody, except now you." At that point she began to sob great big heaving sobs, and tears streamed down her face.

How could she have lived with this for twenty-five years without telling a soul, not even her husband? I knew her husband. He was a prominent businessman in our city. They were both active members in a large, evangelical church in our city. I had given a prolife message at their church years before this office visit.

"I can't teach Sunday School or serve anywhere in the church. I'm not qualified. I have blood on my hands. I helped to kill my own baby!" She grabbed both of my hands in her hands and with a desperate, wild-eyed look in her eyes, she exclaimed, "Dr. Jackson, you've got to help me! What am I going to do?"

What would you tell her? What would you tell this woman in her distress? Would you flinch? Would you look away in embarrassment? No, my brother; no, my sister. You and I must be convinced in our heart of hearts that Jesus Christ can meet every need of the human heart from the unwed mother to our drug addicted brother to our alcoholic neighbor to the porn addict. Once again–Is anything too difficult for God? Is His ear so dull that He cannot hear? Is His arm so short that He cannot save? Of course not!!!

I grasped her hands and looked her in the eye and said plainly and confidently, "Ma'am, the blood of Jesus makes the foulest clean. If He changed the Christian killer Saul into the missionary Paul who planted churches all over Eastern Europe and wrote most of the New Testament books, He can transform you from a baby killer into a Sunday School teacher. There is no sin so great that God will not forgive it. Remember, Moses murdered an Egyptian soldier, yet God used him to lead the children of Israel out of Egypt and up to the Promised Land. Trust me, God can strike a mighty good lick with a crooked stick. In fact, any time He uses any of us, He uses a crooked stick washed clean in the blood of the Lamb."

She stared at my face for the longest time. I could tell she was calculating these truths in her heart and mind. I could see she was struggling internally. Then she began to weep silently again. So I told her a story. I said, "Diana, I had a certain patient in the hospital with pneumonia whose infection was quite severe. I informed him of his diagnosis and that he needed a rather high-powered antibiotic. He nodded, indicating he understood the diagnosis and the treatment.

"However, a few moments later, when I walked back into the room with a large syringe and needle filled with antibiotic medicine, he immediately rebelled saying, 'Oh, no. You are not injecting that into my body!'

"I explained to him again, 'This will help you get better quickly. Without it you may be sick for a long time or even die.'

'I understand that fully and I believe it, but you are not injecting any chemicals into my body.'

"I was quite perplexed. He and I went round and round for a few minutes, but he was adamantly opposed to intravenous injections of medications. I eventually discovered he would take medications by mouth, so we compromised and I gave him those. He eventually got better, albeit slower than he might have otherwise.

"Mrs. Diana, the point of this illustration is my patient had faith in the medication, but he wasn't willing to receive it by IV administration. He wasn't what I call 'receiving-believing.' Likewise, you believe in the ability of God to cleanse us from our sin, but you aren't willing to receive that cleansing for yourself. You are not receiving-believing. The Bible says, 'But as many as received Him, to them He gave the right to become children of God, even to those who believe in His name,' (John 1:12). Becoming a child of God requires receiving and believing. Accepting the forgiveness of God requires receiving and believing. Does that make sense?"

She nodded her head slowly, but I could tell she was having a hard time with this concept. "Do you mind if I make a referral for you to the post-abortion counseling class at the local crisis pregnancy center?" I asked.

"No, I don't mind. I know some of those ladies quite well." So we prayed together and the referral was made. She attended six weeks of post-abortion counseling classes from which she graduated with flying colors. She went on to become a counselor in this same class. I learned later she was teaching a teenage girls' Sunday School class. "Come now, and let us reason together," says the Lord. "Though your sins are as scarlet, they will be as white as snow..." (Isaiah 1:18).

Have you ever had an employee with an attitude? You know what I mean. You ask him to do something and he does it, but begrudgingly. You wonder what you did to him. Did you offend him? Or is he just mad at the world? His attitude is just beneath the surface, not enough to get him fired but enough to make you wonder why you hired him.

Well, I had such an employee. She was a hard worker and efficient, but with an undertone of resistance to authority. She was short and significantly overweight. She fluctuated between really happy and fun to brooding and sullen. She was hard to figure out.

Finally, one day after several years of employment, she asked me if she could speak to me privately. I said, "Sure." So we stepped into an exam room, shut the door, and she shared with me a surprising story.

"Dr. Jackson, when I was fourteen I became pregnant by an older, adult uncle. My mother found out and was furious. She didn't want a family spectacle. At the time abortion was illegal in South Carolina, so we drove to Washington, D.C., where I had an abortion. My mother and I have never discussed the incident again, not even to this day. I was personally devastated, but I was too young to say 'yay' or 'nay' or even think about the consequences. My relationship with my mother has steadily deteriorated ever since. My relationship with all men, even my husband, has been shaky ever since. My mood has been mostly depressed for thirty years. I overeat to compensate emotionally. I can't tell you how that event has negatively impacted my life. I need help desperately."

After a long moment of pondering my next comments, I spoke these words to her in no uncertain terms, "You are the unfortunate victim of the immoral choices of your uncle and your mother. The fallout from their decisions is still affecting your life thirty years later." I said to her confidently, "Jesus can heal all wounds, even thirty-year old wounds. You will have to trust me on this." I then referred her to the crisis pregnancy

123

center post-abortion class as well, where the ladies loved her and counseled with her for many weeks. She left employment at my office shortly after that, and I lost touch with her for a year and half.

Subsequently, she came by my office for a visit. To my embarrassment, I didn't recognize her when she came by. She had lost eighty pounds and did not even resemble her former self. She stood in front of me, talking as if she knew me, but I had no idea who she was. She started laughing and finally identified herself. I nearly fell over. She told me after the healing occurred in the post-abortion class she stopped overeating. She quickly lost the weight. She reconciled with her mother and her husband. Plus, she had the most radiant and pleasant smile on her face. She overflowed with gratitude for the referral to the post-abortion class and for what God had done in her life. A few months later she shared her story with over a thousand people at the crisis pregnancy center's annual fundraising banquet as the CPC featured their post-abortion counseling ministry. Now isn't God good?

The Bible says God can "restore the years the locusts and the canker worm have devoured," (Joel 2:25 KJV). Our God is all about restoration. After all, He has restored you and me to a right relationship with Him through our Lord Jesus Christ. After forty years of abortion on demand, there are many millions of women who have been adversely affected in one way or another by abortion.

One young lady named Breanne, whose interview with Burke and Reardon is recorded in their book *Forbidden Grief,* gives insight into her post abortion distress. She says,

> Most of us who are suffering after our abortions are too ashamed to admit it. The feeling is that you just want to forget about the whole horrible thing. If anyone ever mentioned abortion, I became frozen. Either I would leave

the room or keep quiet. I didn't want anyone
to know what I had done. If I was questioned
about abortion, I didn't want to talk about it
because I was afraid I would start into one
of my uncontrollable crying fits. Those were
moments I reserved for my bedroom where no
one else could see the tears.[1]

Since as many as 50% of post-abortion women hide their
previous abortions from interviewers, researchers have to use
"record based studies that do not rely on surveys of women but
instead look directly at their medical records to assess their
post abortion symptoms."[2] One such study from Finland, using
government records from their government health care system
that covers all health care costs including abortion, revealed
that women who had an abortion "were three times more likely
to commit suicide within a year of their abortion than women
in the general population, and more than six times likely to
commit suicide than women who carried their pregnancy
to term.[3]

Another study from California examined the death records
of low-income women. "Compared to women who delivered,
those who aborted were 154 percent more likely to die from
suicide and 82 percent more likely to die from accidents (which
may be related to suicidal behavior). The higher suicide rates
were most pronounced in the first four years following the
pregnancy outcome."[4]

In 1989 the *Los Angeles Times* surveyed 3,583 people, dis-
covering that 56% of women admitted to a sense of guilt after
abortion and 26% regretted choosing abortion.[5] To once again
quote Burke and Reardon:

If we apply the 56% guilt rate...to the general
population, this is clearly suggestive of a wide-
spread problem. What other medical procedure

has such a high dissatisfaction rate? No one wants to undergo surgery, but one in four heart attack patients regret their decision to undergo heart bypass surgery? Probably not. I suspect this high rate of regret is unique to abortion and is indicative of the psychological conflict that continues to haunt women and men for years after their abortion. [6]

Now I know what the secularists say; you can google "consequences of abortion" and find articles that refute major psychological effects of abortion. It is difficult for researchers to gauge the true effects because women struggle with revealing the truth in their minds and hearts, but hear me well! Just as sin tore at the very heart of King David upon his sinning with Bathsheba, so will the sin of abortion tear at the heart of women and their partners. Sin blinds, sin separates, and sin has consequences!

Please, if you have had an abortion or know someone who has, refer yourself or your friend to your local crisis pregnancy center for post-abortion counseling. Loving Christian women work there who desire to help you find healing and restoration in the Lord, whose name is Jehovah Rafah, the Lord who heals (Exodus 15:26).

RESOURCES (for those who have had an abortion or know someone who has)

Any local CPC–see previous chapter to find one

Crisis Pregnancy: Abortion and Recovery Network

A Partnership between Care Net and American Association of Christian Counselors
http://www.aacc.net/courses/biblical-counseling/crisis-pregnancy

Chapter Ten
Defending All Life–Euthanasia

B efore I sent this book to print, Belgium euthanized via physician-assisted suicide the first terminally ill minor since they lifted age restrictions in 2014.[1] The first country to legalize euthanasia, the Netherlands also "allows mercy killings for children, but only for those twelve and over."[2] Four states — Oregon, Vermont, Washington, and California — legalized physician-assisted suicide by legislation while Montana gives the option by court decision.[3] I have often stated that legalizing abortion put us on a slippery ethical slope. Here are some personal experiences illustrating what happens when we depart from the sanctity of life ethic.

The phone rang at my home in Spartanburg. It was my mom. I could tell she was distressed. "What's the matter, Mom?" I asked.

"It's Aunt Virginia. She's groaning all the time and writhing in bed. She's only semi-conscious. She won't eat or drink. I can't bear to watch her suffer like that."

My great-aunt Virginia had been in a nursing home in Orangeburg, South Carolina, for several years. Sadly, she was now approaching death. Aunt Virginia was a cultured and refined Southern lady with a charming manner and infectious laugh. I loved visiting in her home when I was a small boy. I still wear a family ring every day that she gave me when her husband died. She had no children and my mother was one of her favorite nieces.

"Mom, I'm so sorry. I know that must be hard for you. Are the doctors providing fluids for her?" I already knew the answer.

"No, they have decided to withhold all treatment since she is so near to death."

I suppose I should have been angry or indignant on my aunt's behalf, but I had fought this same battle so many times before that I was resigned to it.

"Mama, providing fluids is not therapeutic or extraordinary care. It is comfort care, basic nurturing care. I recommend providing fluids to all of my institutionalized patients. I don't allow any of my patients in the hospital or nursing home to dehydrate to death. Contrary to what the nursing staff and doctors will tell you, dehydrating to death is a painful way to die. Just look at Aunt Virginia. "

Aunt Virginia lived for several more days before she succumbed to old age and dehydration. Yes, of course, she was going to die anyway, but did she have to die a painful death due to dehydration? Providing fluids is simple, easy, and humane. So what if she lived a few more days? Are we reducing the value of her life to a financial calculation? Are you willing to die a miserable death by dehydration in the end just to save the economy a few miserable dollars? I don't think so!

As I said, this was not the first time I had fought this battle. I managed a nursing home for a number of years when I was first in medical practice. I loved the elderly patients and became quite attached to them. Most of the nurses were devoted to the patients and provided excellent care.

I had one particular patient with dementia who was the father-in-law of a previous governor of South Carolina. His daughter, the governor's wife, visited him often. The patient walked around the facility but did not really recognize anyone. He occasionally became dehydrated, confused, and lethargic. A day or two on fluid supplementation always returned him to his usual baseline status. On one such occasion a night nurse said to me, "He has lived a good, long life. Just let him go."

Because I was a young doctor who had not yet developed the cynicism so common in the medical profession (and by God's grace, I never have), I was startled by her callous disregard for this man's life and the value of his life. I looked at her and replied, "So you want me to intentionally kill the governor's father-in-law by dehydration?"

> *"So you want me to intentionally kill the governor's father-in-law by dehydration?"*

She was the one shocked this time. "Good God, no," she replied.

"Well, that is what you just suggested to me."

She stammered a bit, "Not when you put it that way."

"What way would you like me to put it?"

Indignant, she replied, "You are so crass." She then turned on her heels and stomped off.

I then looked up to heaven and asked, "What did I say?" I ordered fluids for the patient for twenty-four hours; the next day he was up walking around as was his custom. I have seen this same scenario played out in patients who were deemed ready for the mortuary, but when I insisted on basic comfort care, which included fluids, the patient often woke up and resumed his or her normal mental functioning to the amazement, and sometimes indignation, of the medical staff.

Some would accuse me of prolonging the inevitable in my elderly or terminal patients, to which I respond, "When God sends the death angel, there is nothing I can do to forestall His invitation,

> *The answer is medical doctors will fall in the trap of being the purveyors of death rather than the practitioners of life*

but I am committed to not allowing my patients to dehydrate on my watch." I believe that is caring and compassionate medical practice. What happens when medical doctors forsake this time-honored medical practice of providing comfort care? The answer is medical doctors will fall in the trap of being the purveyors of death rather than the practitioners of life just like in Belgium and the Netherlands.

Remember the following:

> The *original* euthanasia program was to "purify" the German race. It was a creation of physicians, *not* Hitler. He simply allowed the use of the tools others had prepared.

> The first gas chamber was designed by professors of psychiatry from twelve major universities. They selected the patients and watched them die. Then they slowly reduced the "price tag" until the mental hospitals were almost empty.

> They were joined by some pediatricians, who began by emptying the institutions of handicapped children in 1939. By 1945 almost 300,000 "pure blood Aryan" Germans had been killed. By then these doctors had so lowered the price tag, that they were killing bed wetters, children with misshapen ears, and those with learning disabilities.[4]

Do you think that was peculiar to the Nazi regime? In my third year of medical school, I walked through the pediatric ICU and found a newborn segregated from all of the other babies with moveable partitions surrounding the bassinet. I inquired regarding his status, and one nurse with distress in her eyes said, "Oh, he's a Down's baby."

I replied, "And what else?"

Sadly, she said, "He has esophageal atresia; his parents have decided they don't want him, so they refused corrective surgery. The medical order states to neglect him until death."

The world stopped. I held onto a table in order to avoid falling into the chasm of nauseating comprehension and shocking incomprehension that clashed in my mind and heart. I finally walked weak and emotionally numb out of the room to ponder how a medical university committed to care for the sick and traumatized could by benign neglect allow an innocent, harmless newborn to die such a wretched death by starvation. This precious little lamb was created by God, but rejected by his parents, and a complicit medical establishment was going to send him back to God prematurely. Of necessity I walked through the pediatric ICU every day observing this travesty. He cried for three days, but after that silence hung in the air. It would have been possible to put a feeding tube in his stomach to provide nutrition, and foster parents would have been easy to find. With a grieving heart on the tenth day, I saw the partitions were gone, and the little Downs boy had gone back to God.

This was in the days before the Americans with Disabilities Act promoted by Ronald Reagan. Such a thing would not happen today (well, I'm not so sure), but it was common before President Reagan began to champion life even for the handicapped. For over thirty-six years I have awakened in the night hearing that little Downs baby crying and tormenting myself, wondering why I didn't just pick that baby up and walk out with him in a blanket. No one was watching him. I really think I could have accomplished it. I was just a young, dumb medical student with poorly formed thinking on life issues. Nevertheless, I knew it wasn't right to let that defenseless little baby die like that when a feeding tube would have preserved his life.

How could his parents be so callous? Was there no other God-fearing, right-thinking person anywhere in the pediatric department of that major medical university? God forgive me for being so passive, for walking by that little baby's crib every day for ten days and not doing anything to rescue him from certain death.

Is what I did all those years ago any different from those of us who drive by the abortion clinics in our cities–passive, nonchalant, unmoved? We know what goes on in those clinics. We know the doctors there kill unborn babies. Yet, we drive by without stopping or praying or grieving. We don't gather our right-thinking Christian friends and make plans to rescue the moms and babies from certain destruction. Why not? Because it's legal? Oh, come on! It used to be legal to own slaves in America. We corrected that heinous wrong. It used to be legal to segregate races in America. We corrected that, also. How long before we make this right?

Our politicians don't see the light until they feel the heat. Pray for them and call them. Write them constantly. Don't let them off the hook. The lives of unborn children hang in the balance. Be a prolife advocate. Don't be passive as I was. I still regret it.

RESOURCES

National Right to Life
512 10th St. NW
Washington, DC 20004
202.626.8800

Susan B. Anthony List
1200 New Hampshire Ave. NW, Suite 750
Washington, DC 20036
202.223.8073

American Life League
P.O.B. 1350
Stafford, VA 22555
540.659.4171

Chapter Eleven

I'm Not A Prophet

"Dr. Jackson, Miss Newman from the CPC is on the phone."

"Put her through." I'm always delighted to talk to Alexia Newman, the director of our local crisis pregnancy center.

"Dr. Jackson, this is Alexia."

"Yes, ma'am. What in the world can I do for you?"

"Would you consider coming to the office for our quarterly volunteer training to teach our volunteers about embryology and abortion techniques?"

Well, this was right up my alley. "I would be delighted. Embryology is fascinating. I would love that. Abortion techniques are droll and depressing, but I can do it. When do you need me?"

Well, this conversation took place over fifteen years ago. I've been privileged to meet and train hundreds of volunteers at the crisis pregnancy centers in Spartanburg and Gaffney, South Carolina, during these years. I usually begin with my prolife journey to illustrate prolife principles and to introduce how the CPC in Spartanburg got started. Then we enjoy talking about the development of the unborn child in the mother's womb.

I begin with something like this.

> We marvel that life begins at conception when
> the sperm and egg join together, usually in

the fallopian tube. The conceptus then begins to multiply into many cells called the morula (mulberry) before implanting three to five days later into the lining of the mother's womb, at which time this little alien being completely takes over! The pregnant mother quickly gains substantial weight and forty percent more fluid volume, grows hair in all manner of strange places, and becomes quite radiant.

This baby has a completely different chromosomal content than that of the mother or the father, twenty-three from mom and twenty-three from dad, which gives the lie to the callous claim from pregnant moms who want to abort their babies when they say, "It's my body; I can do with it what I want to." Well, it is contained within her body, but it is a separate human being with its own unique genetic content as will be made abundantly clear in eight to nine months, when she gives birth.

As soon as they give birth, moms with a normal maternal instinct say things like, "Oh, look at my baby. Isn't he/she precious?" Then they begin to cry tears of joy and relief. I've seen that replayed in the delivery room hundreds of times. That baby was not some meaningless, inanimate part of that mother's body that she could callously dispose of at her whim and caprice. Newborns are precious, beautiful, and loved from the moment their mothers lay eyes on them.

We rejoice when we look at medical photographs of unborn children in the amniotic sac to observe how well developed they are. You can find these under "human embryology" or "human fetal development" on the internet. My favorite photograph is that of a two-month gestational age child plucked from a mother's abdomen during surgery and photographed by Robert Wolfe, then a medical photographer at the University of Minnesota.[1] On March 10, 1970, Dr. Paul E. Rockwell, Director of Anesthesiology, Leonard Hospital, Troy, New York, wrote a letter to the editor of the Albany *Times-Union* about this experience eleven years earlier.[2]

The pregnant mother had unfortunately suffered a ruptured tubal pregnancy. Upon opening her abdomen, the surgeon found the baby in the amniotic sac, still alive, and floating on a pool of blood. He handed the baby to the anesthesiologist, who is holding him between his thumb and forefinger in the picture. The umbilical cord is visible. The anesthesiologist described this tiny human as "being perfectly developed, with long tapering fingers, feet, and toes, ...extremely alive and swam about the sac approximately one time per second, with a natural swimmer's stroke" until the sac broke and the baby died.[3]

How amazing is that! This also makes a lie of the prochoice (pro-death) claim that the unborn child is a meaningless blob of tissue at this stage of development, which is a mantra repeated often in abortion clinics to deceive uncertain clients (ex-employees at abortion clinics have reported this claim; just google "former abortion clinic workers" and read their many stories). I have already told you the story of Abby Johnson, the former director of a Planned Parenthood abortion center, but hear her words. When she assisted the doctor performing that life-changing, ultrasound-guided abortion, she recalled her husband's words:

When you were pregnant with Grace, it wasn't a fetus; it was a baby," Doug had said.

And now it hit me like a lightning bolt: He was right! What was in this woman's womb just a moment ago was alive. It wasn't just tissue, just cells. That was a human baby—fighting for life! A battle that was lost in the blink of an eye. What I have told people for years, what I've believed and taught and defended, is a lie.[4]

At about twenty-one days, the developing baby has a heartbeat, detectable a few days later with third and fourth generation ultrasound machines, which are commonly available today. I remember when my good friend, Dr. John Thornburg, a radiologist, called me on the phone at my office one day in the middle of office hours to report he had just heard for the first time a heartbeat at twenty-eight days (of fetal development) with a new third generation ultrasound using a vaginal probe. He was beside himself with

137

excitement. I couldn't understand a word he said for two to three minutes because of his excitement. We both rejoiced and wondered at this newfound technology and what it might do to turn the tide in the abortion debate.

At forty-nine days, brain wave activity can be measured with sophisticated medical equipment. Now let's ponder that for a moment. If you or I are injured in a serious motor vehicle accident and end up in a neuro-ICU with a severe closed head injury and if, on two consecutive days there is no meaningful neurologic activity, then on the word of two examining physicians (one a neurologist), you or I could be declared legally dead, all life support suspended, and all of our organs donated. Yet, at the other end of the life spectrum, if the little baby in the mother's womb has a heartbeat, brain wave activity, and movement, it has no right to life in America, this "greatest nation on God's green earth" (to quote radio talk show host Michael Medved).[5] Is it, Mr. Medved? Maybe, at one time! What schizophrenic applications of the law! What double standards! What hypocrisy!

By ten weeks, the developing baby has his/her own unique set of fingerprints, forever distinguishing him/her from every other human being that has ever lived on planet earth. The fingerprints you have now were already present at ten weeks of development.

By twelve weeks, almost all organ systems are present and functioning in a rudimentary fashion. Certainly, as the Psalmist affirms, the individual in the womb at this age is profoundly unique and God-ordained. Psalm 139:13-16 says,

For You formed my inward parts; you wove me in my mother's womb. I will give thanks to You, for I am fearfully and wonderfully made. Wonderful are Your works, and my soul knows it very well. My frame was not hidden from You when I was made in secret and skillfully wrought in the depths of the earth. Your eyes have seen my unformed substance, and in Your book were all written the days that were ordained for me when as yet there was not one of them.

If born prematurely at about twenty-four weeks in a city with a modern newborn ICU, greater than fifty percent of these babies will survive in today's world, especially in westernized countries. In normal circumstances, a newly developing life grows rapidly to six–eight pounds, on average, in forty weeks while the mother prospers. Her family and friends remark on her rosy complexion and radiant smile.

What if this was a tumor growing inside her body, not a baby? What if a tumor had grown to six to eight pounds inside her abdomen in nine months time? Why, she would be wasting away, losing weight, and unable to eat with her hair falling out and hollow eyes, and she would be depressed nigh unto death because of the fatal consequences of the malignant growth within her body. No one would say it. They would only think it–"She looks awful. How much longer does she have to live?"

Yet, when a baby grows in her mother's womb, her baby grows larger and faster than any tumor while the mother becomes healthier and more beautiful! How do you explain that? It's the way God made us! It's a God thing! It's a miracle! Can I get a witness? Yes, yes, I see that hand.

Now let's talk about abortion techniques. The most common procedure is the suction aspiration performed between the fifth and twelfth week of gestation, using a powerful suction device twenty-five times more powerful than a home vacuum cleaner. It may be difficult because the cervix is hard and not ready for delivery. The abortionist inserts a hollow, plastic tube, which has a cutting edge on the tip, into the uterus. Suction removes the baby's body and the placenta into a bottle for disposal. Complications, which are rare, include bleeding, infection, cervical laceration, and uterine perforation. Of course, for the baby the procedure is fatal.

The next most common procedure is a dilation and curettage, which is used for thirteen to fifteen weeks gestation and is similar to the aspiration procedure except the abortionist inserts a curette, a looped steel knife, into the uterus with which to cut the baby and the placenta into smaller pieces for easier removal from the uterus. He then scrapes the parts into a basin. Bleeding is profuse. Complications are similar to those above. The effect on the baby is fatal.

Prostaglandin abortions are rarely used anymore except to induce preterm labor in the case of fetal demise during pregnancy. In the 1970s and 1980s, prostaglandin suppositories were given to induce preterm labor. Violent contractions often followed. The preterm babies were sometimes born alive and were disposed of, usually by neglecting them until they died. I have seen this myself [see chapter 1]. Doctors abandoned this procedure due to the high percentage of complications.

Second and third trimester abortions are conducted using the dilatation and evacuation procedure. This procedure involves the live dismemberment of the baby and removal through the cervix. A large forceps is used because the baby's bones and skull are calcified during these trimesters. There is no anesthesia provided for the baby. The abortionist inserts the instrument up into the uterus, seizes a baby body part, and with a twisting motion tears it from the baby's body. This is repeated until all body parts are retrieved, including the skull, which usually has to be crushed.

The nurse's job is to reassemble all of the body parts to assure that nothing has been left behind. This is psychologically devastating to the nursing personnel and also for the doctors, per interviews with nurses and doctors at abortion clinics who have walked away from the abortion industry.[6] You can read the many stories of such medical personnel by googling something like "abortion workers who quit their jobs." Of course, the impact upon the babies is always the same. They end up dead.

Silence hung like a deadly pall over the group of Christian ladies as sadly they digested the information until someone asked, "Dr. Jackson, is this last procedure the same as a partial birth abortion procedure?"

"It's close, but it is not quite the same. A partial birth abortion involves a breech delivery of a live second or third trimester baby. Before the head is delivered, the physician punctures the rear of the skull with a pair of sharp scissors and then suctions out the brains, thereby killing the unborn child. He then delivers an intact but dead baby."

One of the ladies, with tears in her eyes and a trembling lip, asked me, "Why would anybody do that?"

"I'm sorry to tell you that it is done for the sale of fetal parts to research and cosmetic companies."

There was an audible gasp in the room and quiet weeping. "Isn't that illegal?" someone else inquired.

"Yes, ma'am, it is, but mark my words: I'm not a prophet or the son of a prophet, but there is somebody, somewhere still performing this procedure because the sale

I'm not a prophet or the son of a prophet,

of fetal parts is too lucrative for there not to be. You ladies remember I told you that."

Several years later, speaking to a different group of ladies in training, I made the same statement about there being someone in the United States selling fetal parts for financial gain. I told them, "I am not a prophet, nor the son of a prophet," but the financial incentive is too great on the black market for some unscrupulous physician not to be selling fetal parts. I advised them to watch the news.

Within one month in 2015, the Center for Biomedical Progress began releasing their videos exposing Planned Parenthood and their practice of selling fetal parts.[7] As of this writing, twelve videos have now been released.[8] Planned Parenthood is the single largest provider of abortion services in America, providing 323,999 abortions in 2014.[9] Their 2014-2015 annual report indicates that forty-three percent of their budget comes "from payments from Medicaid managed care plans, which are listed as 'Government Health Services Grants and Reimbursements' to reflect the ultimate source of the funds."[10] That's taxpayers' money. That's you and me. Why should we be paying them to kill unborn children and then sell their parts, especially when the most recent Gallup poll reveals that approximately 46% of Americans call themselves prolife (47% prochoice) with 56% of Americans either saying abortion should be completely illegal or legal in only a few circumstances?[11] I am prayerful that our legislators will follow through on their pledge to defund Planned Parenthood.

I have not included the following information in my teaching opportunities at the CPC, but I suppose I should begin to do so. Although abortions have declined around the country, the use of powerful chemicals/drugs, often called "human pesticides," to induce abortions has increased to 22.6% of all abortions since the FDA approved RU-486 in 2000.[13] Composed of two hormones, mifepristone, which essentially starves the baby, and misoprostol, which causes the mother to expel the baby,[14] the drug was initially approved for use on preborn babies up to seven weeks, but in 2016 the FDA approved a new regimen through ten weeks gestation.[15] Additionally, even though the number of abortion clinics has declined, the number of "providers" of these drugs has increased, counting doctors and other "health clinics."[16] As late as June 28, 2016, the Supreme Court set a dangerous precedent by refusing to hear an appeal from prolife pharmacists in Washington state who challenged a state law forcing them to dispense these drugs against their conscience rather than referring clients to other pharmacies.[17]

Before we leave this chapter on embryology, I want to recommend a book to you moms and dads, grandmas and grandpas. It's a great book for discussing life issues. It is by a great theologian–Dr. Seuss. The book is entitled *Horton Hears a Who*. A great movie by the same title exists for those of you with ADD.

The protagonist is an elephant named Horton who hears a plea for help from a microscopic people called the Who (not the rock band). They happen to live on a flower destined for destruction by Horton's contemporaries, who cannot hear their cries for help that only Horton can hear. Horton is derided, scorned, and ridiculed by family, friends, and enemies. Everyone thinks he is crazy and turns against him. Horton encourages everyone in Whoville to make noise so they can be heard. When every last person in Whoville cooperates (because everyone counts), they are finally heard. Their city is spared.

Horton is vindicated. Horton becomes a hero because he is their advocate when no one else cares, when no one else believes, and when no one supports him. Horton concludes the book with this famous statement, "A person is

"A person is a person no matter how small!"

a person no matter how small."[18] Yes! "A person is a person no matter how small!"

What a great prolife message for all of us to remember. Thank you, Dr. Seuss. Thank you, Horton. You and I have a responsibility to teach the next generation to value life and to be prolife advocates. If we don't teach our children and grandchildren, who will? Just as I do my part as a medical doctor training CPC volunteers, we must all do our part training the next generation of prolifers. Horton gives us a good theological start!

Common Abortion Procedures

Taken from the *Intimacy Before Impact Manual*, Chapter 12, Abortion.

Medical Abortion (sometimes known as chemical abortions)

What is medical abortion?	Induced through the use of drugs that are usually taken in pill form, though injections are sometimes used. These medicines work in various ways to bring about the death of the growing embryo or fetus. Medicines which result in the death of an embryo or fetus are known as abortifacients. Though not recognized as "medical abortion," emergency contraception (otherwise known as the "morning-after pill")—sold in the U.S. as *Plan B* or *ella*—has a possible, but unproven, abortifacient effect: altering the endometrium and inhibiting the implantation of a zygote.
When is it used?	In the U.S., the mifepristone/misoprostol regimen is used through nine weeks (63) days of gestation, though the drugs' effectiveness are somewhat diminished after seven weeks (49) days of gestation. Methotrexate/misoprostol are generally used through nine weeks' gestation and sometimes beyond.
What are the side effects?	Pain, cramping, vaginal bleeding, nausea, headache, dizziness, chills, hot flashes, shivering, fatigue, vomiting, diarrhea, and fever.
What are the complications?	Infection, excessive bleeding (hemorrhage) requiring blood transfusion, incomplete abortion (tissue remaining in the uterus), ongoing pregnancy requiring surgical abortion, and—rarely—death.

Type of Regimen	Mifepristone/Misoprostol	Methotrexate/Misoprostol	Misoprostol Only
Description of Procedure	May include two or three visits to the abortion facility. First visit: physical exam confirming gestational age, administration of mifepristone. Second visit (two days later): the second chemical (misoprostol) given.	Requires three or four visits to the abortion facility. First visit: physical exam confirming gestational age, administration of methotrexate, and a dose of misoprostol with directions for self-administration within a few days. Second visit: about a week later, additional exam to determine if a gestational sac is observed. If not, the abortion is considered complete. If yes, another dose of misoprostol will be given, to be followed by a third visit. If a heartbeat is observed, vacuum aspiration will be recommended. If the gestational sac is present, but the embryo has died, a fourth follow-up appointment will be scheduled for three weeks later.	Optimally misoprostol pills are administered vaginally near the cervix. Placing the pills in the mouth, between the cheek and gum, or under the tongue is also effective. A second dose is given 24 hours later. Uterine cramping and vaginal bleeding usually start within hours. Bleeding typically lasts 7–10 days. Many women will pass blood clots, and the embryo can sometimes be observed in the expelled tissue and blood.
Other Notes	Mifepristone is also known as RU-486 or Mifeprex. Misoprostol is also known as Cytotec.	Using this regimen, abortion is not considered complete until the gestational sac is expelled or has been removed via vacuum aspiration. Currently this regimen is not FDA-approved.	This misoprostol-only regimen is not approved by the FDA in the U.S. It is only approved by the FDA for use in conjunction with mifepristone.

Surgical Abortion

What is surgical abortion?	A form of abortion in which the embryo is removed from the uterus using surgical methods.			
Other Notes	· The cervix will need to be dilated in order for the clinician to gain access to the uterus. To dilate the cervix, dilators (made of stainless steel or plastic) or osmotic dilators—either synthetic or natural (known as laminaria)—may be used. A speculum will be inserted into the vagina in order for the cervix to be observed and to provide access for the dilators and other instruments. The woman will likely receive medicine for the pain and may be offered a sedative to relax and calm her. · Abortions using a handheld syringe are known as manual vacuum aspiration, or MVA. Abortions using an electric pump are known as electric vacuum aspiration, or EVA.			

Type of Method	Vacuum Aspiration	Dilation and Curettage (D&C)	Dilation and Evacuation (D&E)	Instillation (or saline)
When is it used?	Generally performed until the 14th week of gestation.	Generally performed until the 14th week of gestation	Generally performed after the 14th week of gestation	Although rare, generally performed in the second and third trimesters.
What is it?	A method in which the contents of the uterus, including the embryo, are removed using a plastic or metal cannula attached to a suction device.	A method in which the contents of the uterus, including the embryo/fetus, are removed using a curette and vacuum aspiration.	Same as a D&C but the main difference is the use of forceps. If forceps are used, the procedure is called a D&E.	A chemical solution is injected through the abdomen of the pregnant woman into the amniotic sac, the membranes that surround and protect the developing embryo.
What are the side effects?	Pain, cramping, vaginal bleeding, diarrhea, and the nausea and vomiting generally associated with anesthesia use.	Vaginal bleeding, cramps, nausea, vomiting, and feeling faint.	Vaginal bleeding, cramps, nausea, vomiting, and feeling faint.	Pain, cramping, vaginal bleeding, fever, nausea, headache, and dizziness.
What are the complications?	Infection, excessive bleeding (hemorrhage), cervical injury, incomplete abortion, uterine perforation, anesthetic complications, and ongoing pregnancy.	Infection, blood clots, injury to the cervix or uterine lining, perforation of the uterus, hemorrhage (moderate to severe internal bleeding), and incomplete abortion.	Infection, blood clots, injury to the cervix or uterine lining, perforation of the uterus, hemorrhage (moderate to severe internal bleeding), and incomplete abortion.	Hemorrhage, infection, accidental injection of solution into the mother's bloodstream, and damage to the uterus during the injection procedure.

This information was taken from *Abortion Explained* (Grand Rapids: LIFE International, 2012).

Used by permission of LIFE International

RESOURCE

Intimacy Before Impact (a volunteer training manual) can be ordered from:

Life International
73 Ransom Avenue NE
Grand Rapids, Michigan 49503

Chapter Twelve

Rescuing The Perishing

I was standing by the door of our prison cell when the food slot at the bottom of the door opened. A voice came from the food slot, "Pssst... hey, come here. I need to talk to somebody."

I quickly got on my knees and looked at two dark brown eyes peering at me through the food slot. I recognized them as belonging to one of the trusties at the Greenville County Detention Center who delivered our meals. He looked up and down the halls knowing surveillance cameras could easily see him on his knees looking and talking through the slot in the door, which was forbidden. Whatever his business, he needed to talk fast before the detention officers came and ran him off.

"What's your name?" he asked.

"My name is Robert Jackson."

"Oh, yeah, you're the doctor."

"Yes, how do you know?"

"Everybody in here knows that a doctor and a bunch of preachers got busted at the abortion clinic. We think that stinks. We all deserve to be here. Y'all don't deserve it. It ain't right. But that's not what I'm here for. I've got to get right with God. Can you help me?"

"Can I help you? Did the Apostle Paul like to share his testimony? Sure, I can help you. Tell me. Why do you need to get right with God?"

"I've been a thief all of my life. I've been abusing drugs since I was thirteen. I've got a girl and two kids. I need to do right by them. I've been talking to some of the pastors in the kitchen. I compare my life to theirs and my life is a wreck. I've just got to get right with God."

Miraculously, no officers appeared. In the next ten to fifteen minutes, I reviewed with him the basics of the gospel message. Obviously, God had already prepared his heart. So kneeling at the food slot at the Greenville Detention Center, I had the privilege to lead this repentant young man to Christ. It was obviously worth a few days in the slammer. That group of pastors and laymen led nineteen men to Christ during those few days of jail ministry!

As you can tell, my best teaching method is by telling stories of events that occurred in my life. My sons-in-law think it's the coolest thing when I begin a story, "When I was in prison..." Actually, I was arrested multiple times when I was praying or rescuing at the abortion clinic, but I was in prison only three times. I don't say that proudly; I say this with deep sadness that in America we "call evil good and good evil," and we "substitute darkness for light and light for darkness..." (Isaiah 5:20). I'm ashamed that in America, when God-fearing, right-thinking people pray at abortion mills where innocent unborn children are murdered and everyone knows it, that the legal system imprisons the pastors and laymen and protects the baby killers (abortion doctors).

"Woe to those who make unjust laws, to those who issue oppressive decrees, to deprive the poor of their rights, and withhold justice from the oppressed of my people, making widows their prey and robbing the fatherless," (Is. 10:1-2 NIV).

So I was asked, "How can one justify breaking the law like that, repeatedly?" Trust me. It was not done lightly. It was only with a great deal of prayer and forethought. Many of these pastors had never even had a speeding ticket. They were crushed in their spirits to be arrested by the very officers they prayed for weekly, that God would protect them in the line of duty. They were brokenhearted that our society would angrily take the side of the abortionist under the guise of upholding the law of man (trespassing) while ignoring the higher law of God, "You shall not murder," (Exodus 20:13). Ultimately, when we distill the issue down to its barest essence, it boils down to:

1) We knew the clear instruction of the word of God to "rescue those being led away to death..." (Proverbs 24:11 NIV).

2) We knew where the killing of the unborn was happening and when. The scripture made it plain that we could not claim ignorance in the presence of God and get away with it. "If you say, 'But we knew nothing about this,' does not he who weighs the heart perceive it? Does not he who guards your life know it? Will he not repay each person according to what he has done?" (Proverbs 24:12 NIV)

3) We knew the divine laws of God had a higher claim on our lives than the temporal laws of man. More than this, there were many scriptural examples of biblical heroes who chose to obey God rather than man whom God honored for their obedience.

> *We knew the divine laws of God had a higher claim on our lives than the temporal laws of man.*

For example, Daniel's three friends — Shadrach, Meshach, and Abednego — defied the king's command to bow down to the golden image of himself that he had erected. Ultimately thrown into the fiery furnace for their civil disobedience, they chose death rather than violate their consciences or disobey God. Their emphatic response to the king was, "Oh, Nebuchadnezzar, we do not need to defend ourselves before you in this matter. If we are thrown into the blazing furnace, the God we serve is able to save us from it, and He will rescue us from your hand, O king. But even if He does not, we want you to know, O king, that we will not serve your gods or worship the image of gold you have set up," (Daniel 3:16-18 NIV). Supernaturally, God rescued these courageous young men, and Nebuchadnezzar was so astonished that he himself praised the Lord. "Praise be to the God of Shadrach, Meshach, and Abednego, who has sent His angel and rescued His servants," (Daniel 3:28 NIV).

Daniel experienced the same conflict a little later. This time the king was Darius. His administrators were jealous of Daniel, so they enticed the king to create a new law saying anyone who worshiped any god except for him for thirty days would be thrown into the lion's den. This appealed to Darius' vanity, and he readily agreed to it. You know the rest of the story. Daniel did not even have to think about it. He knew his obligation was to the higher law of God. He went to his home "just as he had done before," got down on his knees, and prayed toward Jerusalem (Daniel 6:10 NIV). His enemies reported him immediately, and he was thrown into the lions' den. God supernaturally rescued him from the lions. The king hurried the next morning to see if Daniel had survived. Daniel's answer to the king's anguished query was, "Oh king, live forever! My God sent His angel and He shut the mouths of the lions. They have not hurt me, because I was found innocent in His sight nor have I ever done any wrong before you, O king," (Daniel 6:21-22 NIV). Here we see a biblical hero who was found innocent in the sight of God, who was vindicated by God, and who was rescued by God despite the fact that he disobeyed the laws of man.

In the New Testament, the Pharisees commanded Peter and John not to speak any longer in the name of Jesus. They were concerned about the number of people converted to this new way of thinking. They thought they had extinguished Christ's teaching by crucifying Him. Now His followers were preaching His resurrection and thousands were becoming His disciples. They thought they had the authority to squelch free speech. All law-abiding Jews who did not wish to be cast out of the temple obeyed every edict of the Pharisees.

When commanded to speak no further in the name of Jesus, knowing that the Pharisees could cast them out of the temple and could have them arrested and beaten, Peter and John answered in Acts 4:19 (NIV), "...Judge for yourselves whether it is right in God's sight to obey you rather than God. For we cannot help speaking about what we have seen and heard." These men chose to obey the higher law of God rather than the arbitrary, religious edict of man, although they represented the highest law in the land other than the Roman military tribunal.

As we contemplated trespassing on the abortion clinic property to block entrance to the clinic with our physical presence, our pastors were terribly conflicted. As I said, some of them had never even had a parking or speeding ticket. They were squeaky clean. One of them rode with the police officers as a police force chaplain. We were on their side. We were the good guys. All we had planned to do was sit in front of the abortion clinic and pray, but the idea of breaking any law did not sit well with any of us. Nevertheless, the awareness that unborn children were being killed in that clinic caused us untold grief. Knowing God commanded us to rescue those being led away to death caused us a serious moral conflict.

Finally, one pastor stood up and said, "Brothers, we all looked down upon the German Christians who failed to come to the rescue of the Jews in Nazi Germany. They sang louder in church to drown out the cries of the Jews as they went by in the cattle cars on the way to concentration camps. They knew what was happening, and they hid behind their religious ceremonies. They feared the Nazis and the concentration camps more than they feared God.[1] All we have to fear is a trespassing ticket. I, for one, am not going to let another baby die in that clinic even if the consequences are much greater. I have to do what I have to do. Obviously, the legal establishment in this country is not going to do anything to protect the unborn.

"Brothers, it is up to you and me. I can't stand the thought of succeeding generations looking back on us and saying, 'Why didn't those Christian pastors do something? Didn't they know they were killing babies in the abortion clinics?' Even if I am the only one, I'm going to sit by the door of that clinic this Saturday morning!!"

That did it. Numerous pastors and laymen agreed to participate. That led to several peaceful, prayerful rescue attempts at the two abortion clinics in Greenville, South Carolina, the city adjacent to my hometown of Spartanburg. On one occasion, my medical partner and I were arrested along with about forty pastors on a freezing cold Saturday morning with sleet falling all around us. The clinic was effectively closed for the entire day. Because we declined to post bond, all of us were sentenced to ten days in the detention center.

On another occasion, 800-plus people lined up to pray on a public sidewalk across the street from one of the abortion clinics in Greenville. There were no signs. There was no talking. All we did was pray silently. The magistrate and sheriff of Greenville County were so supportive of the abortion clinics and so agitated by our prolife activity, they decided to arrest all 800 people. About one hour into our four-hour prayer vigil, school buses arrived and officers began to arrest people for praying on the public sidewalk. We asked them, "Why?" They said we were picketing without a permit! Initially, we were incredulous; then we began to laugh ourselves silly. Then we simply said, "Ok, everybody get on the buses. We will pray downtown."

The only problem was they didn't have enough personnel to process 800 people in a timely fashion. After a few hours they realized the foolishness of trying to do so, so they just told everybody to go home. Half of us prayer warriors were still praying on the sidewalk, and half were praying at a large downtown auditorium where they were being processed. Anti-life officials will do the most foolish things to vent their anger at peaceful, praying people. "Why are the nations in an uproar, and the peoples devising a vain thing?" (Psalm 2:1)

Back to the Greenville Detention Center–on another occasion I served my time later than the rest of the group because I did not want to be out of my medical office at the same time as my partner, Dr. Bailes, who was arrested at the same time I was. Both Marty Clary, a pitcher for the Atlanta Braves, and I served our time later than the rest. We actually served our time about six months later to allow Marty to finish his baseball season.

On Sunday, while resting between kitchen duty (Marty and I were assigned to wash pots and clean tables between meals), I received a phone call from one of the Pastors for Life, Michael Cloer, then pastor of Siloam Baptist Church in Powdersville, South Carolina. He said, "Brother Robert, just wanted you to know that when we conducted our rescue last year, a young lady from Greenwood, South Carolina, saw all the commotion and decided to turn around and go home. She ultimately decided to deliver her baby and make an adoption plan. A young couple from my church adopted that baby. We dedicated her baby to the Lord in our morning worship service today. I thought that would encourage you and Marty."

I was surprised and speechless. I was overcome with emotion. Through my tears, I mumbled my thanks. I went back to my cellblock, where Marty and I bunked with nineteen other guys. I found Marty and told him the news. We stared at each other for a few minutes; then Marty said, "It was really worth it, wasn't it? The arrest, the humiliation, being fingerprinted, being in here for a week..." I thought about it for a long moment.

A close family member had told me I was the biggest fool he had ever met for participating in the rescue. Another doctor had warned me it would ruin my reputation and my medical practice. (In fact, my reputation in the Christian community soared and my medical practice prospered). My, how God is faithful when His children are obedient. I looked at Marty and we both began to tear up.

I said, "I suspect there were others who changed their minds that we don't even know about. But even if this little girl was the only one, it really is worth it." Then we began to laugh out loud and to slap each other on the back, praising the Lord for all we were worthwhile the nineteen other guys in our new Cell Block B Bible study group looked at us in astonishment.

Chapter Thirteen

A Father's Love

Rebecca Wall slumped in my exam room chair with tears streaming down her face. "How am I going to tell my daddy? He's going to kill me." The mascara ran down both cheeks in a dark-stained river, desperation evident in her eyes, wet from uncontrollable heaving sobs. I had just confirmed for this divorced, unwed patient that she was pregnant.

I had known her family for a long time. Her parents were missionaries in Haiti and longtime patients. Her dad was a pastor, evangelist, and church planter. Really, he was a prophet who did not trifle with foolishness or sin. He had planted over twenty churches in northern Haiti in twenty-five plus years of ministry. A self-taught nurse who ran a health clinic on their mission compound, his wife was so good and so compassionate that the Haitians preferred her over the Haitian-trained doctors five miles closer down the road.

I experienced the privilege of serving side-by-side with her parents on multiple occasions in northern Haiti, and our church built two medical clinic buildings on their mission compound. We were heavily invested financially and emotionally in their ministry and in their family. I loved this family deeply.

On one occasion, I arrived at their mission compound to find Rebecca's father seriously burned from head to toe from an explosion in a trash fire. I tended to second and third degree burns on his face, torso, and extremities every day for ten days. Thankfully, I had brought with me everything I needed for just such an emergency. He painfully recuperated over a long time with no infection or scarring. If I had not chosen that particular week for my mission trip, he probably would have required an airlift to the States for adequate therapy.

Rebecca, though, was a rebel. She had been dismissed from Bible school some years previously. She had lived with my family for a short period, where she prospered spiritually until she met a young man. After a whirlwind romance, she married him against our advice and without her parents' approval. That marriage lasted less than two years. Her pastor father took her back in — depressed, embarrassed, and divorced. That is a father's love.

Now this rebel girl had become involved with another man, a married man; she found herself pregnant and unmarried, caught like a bird in a cage. Like the woman caught in adultery, brought to Jesus, and thrown at His feet by the hypocritical Pharisees, she was about to be thrown at the feet of her missionary/pastor/prophet father and exposed for what she really was in front of God and everybody!

As she sat there trembling and sobbing, I offered this proposition, "Rebecca, do you want me to tell your daddy?"

With desperate eyes welling up again with tears, she cried, "Oh, my gosh, Dr. Jackson, would you do that? I can't. I know I can't."

"All right. I'll ask him to come to the office to speak to me tomorrow, but you will have to promise me that you will speak to him the next day," I offered.

"Okay, I can do that. Thank you, Dr. Jackson, thank you." Then she hugged my neck until it almost broke in two.

Two days later her pastor father sat in the same chair where Rebecca sat, and I told him his youngest child, his beloved daughter, was pregnant and not married. Worse than that, she was pregnant by a married man with whom she had no future. His usually strong persona crumbled before my eyes and he wept silently, slowly clenching and unclenching his fists. That was a hard day for both of us as I put my arms around his neck and we wept together. I said nothing. What could I say of any significance?

After a few long moments alone with his thoughts, he thanked me for my kindness, and he promised he would deal kindly with his daughter. He left my office — a broken man.

The next day I called Rebecca to ask her how things had gone with her dad. Through her tears, she told me her dad called her and asked her to come to his house to speak to him. She said, "Dr. Jackson, I went there with fear and trembling, but my father met me at the door. He threw his arms around my neck, and he said, 'Rebecca, I want you to know I love you forever. I want you to know I will love this baby. I want you to break the lease on your apartment and move back home with me and your mother.' That's all he said about it." Wow, now, that's a father's love.

The road for Rebecca was not easy. She experienced pressure from the baby's father to abort him on numerous occasions. She was a single mom after she delivered a precious little boy whom she named Micah. Finding good employment proved difficult. Statistics prove that being an unwed mother is the surest path to poverty in America. She learned that the hard way. If her parents had not allowed her to live in their home and eat their food, she could have been living in a shelter or under a bridge. Her father's generosity proved a father's love.

You and I were rebels, just like my friend Rebecca. You and I have disappointed our Heavenly Father in more ways than we can count. We have been unfaithful to our Lord Jesus Christ. Just as Rebecca thought it would be a fearful thing to face her preacher daddy, it is surely a fearful thing for unrepentant sinners to fall into the hands of the living God.

Our God is a holy God and His "eyes are too pure to look on evil," (Habakkuk 1:13 NIV). He is the righteous judge of all the nations, to whom we must all give account, before whom we must all stand, before whose gaze all the heavens and earth flee away. He Himself is the absolute standard of righteousness against which standard all men's lives will be judged. In His presence, the cherubim fall down and cry, "Holy, Holy, Holy." The twenty-four elders fall down and cast their crowns at His feet in worship. In His presence, you and I, my friend, will be undone, totally exposed, speechless and, like Rebecca, frightened out of our wits if we stand there apart from our Father's love, if we stand there without Jesus, the Father's only Son and our only Advocate.

Hear me clearly. I am weeping as I write this, because my pastor friend's love and unconditional acceptance of his daughter Rebecca so clearly illustrates the love and acceptance of our Heavenly Father that I cannot write this with dry eyes. Paul tells us in Romans 8:1, "There is therefore now no condemnation for those who are in Christ Jesus." There is the catch. We must be in Christ Jesus. We must be spiritually born again.

My friend had the grace and love to accept his sinful and rebellious daughter without anger or reservation because he had the love of God in his heart. He was in Christ Jesus. He had himself experienced forgiveness and God's grace in his own life. How could he not extend the same to his own daughter? It would have been the height of hypocrisy not to have done so. That is not how the Christian life works. Jesus taught us to pray, "Father, forgive me of my transgressions even as I forgive those who have sinned against me," (my paraphrase of Matthew 6:12).

My pastor friend understood this all too well. More than that, his heart was full of a father's love and compassion, just like our Heavenly Father loves us. The scripture tells us that Jesus looked on the crowds that followed Him and His heart

160

"felt compassion for them, because they were distressed and downcast like sheep without a shepherd," (Matthew 9:36). That is the Savior's love.

The Heavenly Father knows your rebellion and mine. He knows our weakness and our frailty and that we are but dust. He knows our hearts are prone to wander, prone to be unfaithful, and prone to lust after other lovers. Knowing all of this, "...God so loved the world, that He gave His only begotten Son, that whoever believes in Him should not perish, but have eternal life," (John 3:16). My friend, that is the Father's love.

Chapter Fourteen

Loving The Orphans

M y eldest daughter, Rachel, came to me several years ago and said, "Dad, you know if abortion is made illegal, many more children will be in foster care. Trevor and I have a heart for abandoned, lost children and are applying to be foster parents."

Even though my mind raced to ponder the many difficult stories I had heard regarding fostering and adoption, I looked at my daughter without hesitation and replied, "Yes, and the church needs to be willing to be the hands and feet of Jesus by taking in these children." I knew clearly the biblical mandate–to take care of the orphans and the widows.

Every day people labor tirelessly to eliminate abortion in the United States–volunteering at crisis pregnancy centers, lobbying congressmen to pass prolife legislation, and providing education on prolife issues. In the meanwhile others work to provide meaningful and viable options to abortion that come in many different flavors, including caring for foster children. Statistics on foster children taken from The AFCARS (Adoption and Foster Care Analysis and Reporting System) Report by the Administration for Children and Families under the U.S. Department of Health and Human Services website reveal the number of children in foster care grew from 404,878 in 2010 to 415,129 in 2014 in the United States with forty-four percent at six years old or less.[1]

So here we are five years later, and in this short period Rachel and Trevor have fostered fifteen children. Currently, they care for two children full time in addition to their own three biological ones. Let us hear Rachel's heart.

RACHEL

Last year I sent out a Christmas newsletter stating what a challenging year 2015 had been. Well, I'm 100% convinced that God saw what I wrote, and He laughed and laughed and laughed and said, "Just wait to see what I have in mind for this year!!!" Now I don't believe God laughed out of sarcasm or unkindness but out of a heart of love for me because He knew what my own heart needed to understand. He knew already the lessons He wanted to teach me.

I now call myself a "trauma mama" (I have several similar women in my life whom I deeply respect who are "trauma mamas"), and I'm barely 32 years old. It is because the year brought teenage boyfriends, cigarettes, alcohol, name-calling, razor cutting, deceit, and lying. It is because the year brought destruction to walls, decor, and beds, sleepless nights, and food and sugar cravings by a child plus extreme separation anxiety, anger, anger, and more anger, fear, disappointment, and hate. It is because a child held onto a school table leg for dear life because he got upset; his fears escalated and he immediately went into "survival mode." Even worse, one child tried to light things on fire from my gas burner store. He required constant one-on-one supervision because he was a hair-trigger bomb ready to explode. He was so underdeveloped emotionally and physically, it was like having a 100-pound toddler with a lightning quick fuse.

What sort of life experiences prepared me for such? I can tell you these behaviors are outside of my box. My early years could best be described as the quintessential, idyllic childhood. I received piano, violin, and vocal lessons, playing the violin for an orchestra and singing in choruses plus I rode horses at my leisure and read novels every day. I attended a prestigious college and was formally educated in biological sciences, literature, and music. My mother devoted her life to educating, nurturing, and discipling her nine children. My father exemplified faithfulness, integrity, a strong work ethic, and was absolutely besotted with his children. Even when life was difficult for my parents with two special needs children, who experienced multiple surgeries, multiple life-threatening situations, and years of therapies, they never let us children feel the stress of my brothers' problems, and they shouldered the responsibility of caring for them with aplomb. Regardless of my brothers' less than optimum capabilities, both cognitively and physically, we accepted these boys into our family with open arms and lavished them with affection and adoration. Never were two special needs boys more cherished or valued. They probably still don't realize there is anything different about them.

In addition to loving these boys, I watched my parents love the unlovely, welcoming former prisoners, adulterers, thieves, liars, the homeless and much more into our home. We fed them, clothed them, housed them, bought them cars, and found them jobs. We children were all engaged in the relationships and accepted these relationships as a normal way of life. Likewise, my husband Trevor watched his parents take in wandering lost souls from pregnant teenage moms to four foster children, who were eventually adopted by his sister.

Why do I tell you all of this? Did any of this prepare me for foster parenting? Yes, yes, it did! God gave me a heart of gratefulness. I can look back at my life and be grateful for my childhood, and, consequently, from a grateful heart I want the same experience for all children. Every child should be raised where there is joy, peace, and tranquility. From caring for my brothers and the unlovely, my life foundation was strong and sure. My heart was full of compassion for humankind and longed to make a difference. The component of compassion entrenched in the core of my being drove me into the perilous waters of harboring children who have disappointment, destruction, and defeat embedded in their hearts.

This compassion met rejection head on. I came brutally face-to-face with the ugly consequences of the physical, verbal, and mental abuse and rejection dispensed by the very parents who should have loved these children the most. I witnessed the painful and tumultuous drama that flows from broken and completely lost hearts. Then eventually, I experienced a pain I had never known because I encountered the deep hurt of rejection myself early in 2016. I found my best advice, my loving care, and my sacrifices thrown away by a foster child making dreadful, life-altering choices, and I found myself with a heavy heart, intense pain, and extreme anger towards this child. It rocked my very core. It tested my identity of who I am. It threatened my commitment to compassionate work, and even caused me to question my God and my faith.

After days of struggling with God and myself, I began to ponder how Jesus felt when the world rejected Him and hung Him on a cruel Roman cross. John 1:10-11 says, "He was in the world, and the world was made through Him, and the world did not know Him. He came to His own, and those who were His own did not receive Him." Christ accepted freely and completely the weight of His cross; plus, He forgave the ones who placed it on Him–you and me. It was an injustice. He had done nothing wrong. He had only given His best advice, loving care, and ultimately His very life as a sacrifice for all of us, and He was rejected. Yet, He forgave. Surely, if He forgave me, I could forgive this child! If He loved me so much, I could love this child!

I also remembered a commitment I had made earlier after reading a quote from the developmental psychologist, Urie Bronfenbrenner, which goes like this, "In order to develop normally, a child requires progressively more complex joint activity with one or more adults who have an irrational emotional relationship with the child. [In other words] Somebody's got to be crazy about that kid. That's number one. First, last and always."[2] I had decided I would be crazy about every kid who came into my home, and this kid was no different. I had decided it didn't matter what behaviors a child displayed; there was a beating heart underneath it all that desperately needed the security of a mother's unconditional love and acceptance.

So I chose to be crazy about this kid! I gave my pain of rejection over to Jesus, and I began to have a greater understanding of the rejection these children have experienced. Just like Jesus said (in so many words), I now very intentionally and frequently say, "I love you and I am not rejecting you. You are accepted and you belong." The world, like Jesus' disciples, often devalues and rejects little children. However, Jesus, with open arms, beckons little children to come unto Him, saying, "... of such is the kingdom of God" (Mark 10:13-16). Even if their actions have consequences, I always reassure them they are loved and accepted. For sure, in my experience, creating a safe, nurturing home with a strong sense of acceptance and belonging–regardless of behavior–has taken care of most behaviors. Thankfully, we are on an upward curve with this particular child, and she has become a joy to have around, voluntarily helping with chores around our home and helping us stay organized. Her favorite week of the year is our summer camp full of swimming, boating, games, singing, and Bible teaching for 40 plus foster kids sponsored by Royal Family Kids in Wasilla, Alaska. Through RFK we also sponsor a monthly mentoring program and hope to expand our camp program.

With another child (the one who started fires and held on to table legs, who was continually suspended from school for aggression, and who had been in 20 different foster homes, the last in which he caused $2,400 worth of damage), I immediately started applying crazy love, and almost overnight he began sleeping through the night (albeit after incrementally decreasing amounts of hugs); he stopped stealing sugar, stopped overeating, and by six weeks, he was almost 100% compliant, listening and obeying almost all the time. The transformation has been dramatic, rapid, and astonishing. We still have many things to work on, but he has come so, so far. Sadly, there are so many children just like him, just like him!!! They just need crazy love!!

I say all of this to say, "Do not be afraid. Do not be afraid! Love wins! Love wins!" Yes, fostering is difficult, very difficult, but do not be afraid! Jehovah Jireh, the God who provides, will meet your every need. He is our greatest resource, and He has many rich lessons to teach you and me about Himself, about loving other people. Christ made a difference in my life. He gave me hope–for an abundant life and eternal life. He desires to use us in the lives of children to make a difference, to give them hope, and to love them unconditionally–just like He does you and me.

* * *

Latretia is sixteen years old and is living in her sixth foster home in two years. She was taken from her parents due to drugs in the home and sexual abuse by an uncle. Admittedly, some of the frequent transfers were due to her acting out behavior, but what teenage girl wouldn't act out under these circumstances? Latretia carries a very large suitcase-like bag everywhere she goes. She even sleeps with it at night. When asked about it, she responded:

> The DSS workers came to my first foster home to get me when I was in school. When they picked me up and transferred me to another foster home in another city, I protested that all of my belongings were at home. It didn't matter to them. They were in a hurry. My only connection to my real family was some pictures I had at the foster home. I also had a few clothes, some makeup, and some jewelry. I lost it all that day. I never saw it again. So I

keep everything I own in this big bag. It never
leaves my sight. I never know when DSS is
going to come and move me to another place.
I'm always prepared.

That sad story was shared with Carmen Gardner's
daughter, Karsyn Blanton of Gaffney, South Carolina. Neither
woman could imagine the emotional distress of being moved
that many times and losing all of one's possessions. Moved
to action by Latretia's story, they conceived the idea of creating care packages for young girls in the foster care program
called "Bags of Beauty" based on a verse in Song of Solomon,
"You are altogether beautiful, my love; there is no flaw in you,"
(Song of Solomon 4:7 ESV).

Each bag contains feminine products, toothbrushes,
hairbrushes, hair products, cosmetics, nail polish, etc. Their
goal is to help girls in foster care feel pretty and clean, and
to help them feel good about themselves. The bags also
include Bibles, journals, pens, and a card with Carmen and/
or Karsyn's phone number so the girls can call for counseling. The idea caught on quickly in her community, and
soon items were donated by businesses in town, even extra
nice bags with the words "Bags of Beauty" monogrammed
on their sides. Karsyn and her friends help pack all of the
bags; then they are given to the Guardian Ad Litem program
in Cherokee County (SC) for distribution. As of this writing,
you can find them on Facebook; other communities offer similar bags to girls in the foster care systems in their cities.

When I look at the number of children in the foster care
system in America and the number of evangelical churches in
America, I wonder why any children are stuck in the system
at all. I realize there are difficult children in the system, but
who better to handle difficult children than God-fearing,
spirit-filled Christian people who are full of the Holy Ghost
and wisdom?

When David Platt, author of *Radical* (a book I highly recommend and use in my discipleship groups) and current president of the International Mission Board of the Southern Baptist Convention, pastored the Church at Brook Hills in Birmingham, Alabama, he challenged his church to foster or adopt all of the foster care children in their huge city. He contacted the Department of Human Resources and discovered the need for 150 families. His church people took the challenge, and they emptied the foster care system in Birmingham.[2] That could, and probably should, happen all over the United States. I'm just saying!

RESOURCES

Royal Family Kids
3000 W. MacArthur Blvd., Suite 412
Santa Ana, CA 9204
714.438.2494
royalfamilykids.org

Bags of Beauty
See Facebook
Gaffney, SC
864.487.0145

Chapter Fifteen

Entertaining Angels Unaware

No prolife book is complete without a discussion of adoption. Indeed, every prolife rally has signs that say "Adoption, Not Abortion," or "Choose Adoption, Not Abortion." Why is this? It is because before 1973 most women caught in unplanned pregnancies made adoption plans (often staying out of sight for six months), or they bore the shame and kept their children. Illegal abortions were available, but mainly for the wealthy.

In my attempt to discover exactly how many couples were out there wanting to adopt a baby, I learned no solid, consistent statistics exist. How does one survey every couple who would like to adopt? You know such couples and I know couples, but no one has officially asked them in order to collect statistics for some article or research. One source stated one to two million couples/individuals are currently waiting to adopt while another source stated four to five million couples. I suspect there is a correct number somewhere in between. With this many couples wanting to adopt a baby, why do we abort 1.1 million children every year in this country? The prochoice side lies when they say abortion solves the problem of "unwanted children." The mother may reject her child, but there are those one to five million other parents desperately praying for a baby. There is no such thing as an unwanted child in America.

"Why can't we love them both?" asked Dr. John Wilke, past president of National Right to Life.[1] Why can't we love and support mother and unborn child? Why do we have to abort the baby? Someone wants every child and no mother needs to live with remorse and regret all of her life. America need not exist with a national guilty conscience. Collectively, we can do better than this.

None of us who were raised with parents of our own will ever understand the desperation with which an orphaned child prays for someone–anyone–to adopt him out of the orphanage or foster system into a real home situation. Likewise, we cannot comprehend the eagerness with which an orphan anticipates the day when adoptive parents arrive to take him away from an orphanage and into a home — a real home, a real family.

None of us, as Christians, really comprehend what it means that we have been adopted as sons through Jesus Christ into the family of God. We intellectually accept that as true, but we really don't live as if it is true. We are royalty, but we live as commoners. "In love He predestined us to be adopted as sons through Jesus Christ according to His pleasure and will," (Ephesians 1:5). This was based entirely on God's initiative and good will toward you and me, altogether apart from any merit of our own. This spiritual adoption was extended to us entirely by His grace (unmerited favor). How amazing is that!

I have friends and patients who adopt children or take children into their homes as foster children for a variety of different reasons. As I observe their unselfish dedication to their children, I think of God's sacrificial love for us and His willingness to adopt us into His family, not because we deserve it, but just because He is good. He is that kind of a God. He is good and kind and merciful. What an awesome God! What a wonderful Savior! Praise God for the following stories!

As I researched information on adoptions, I met two delightful, energetic young ladies, whose vision became reality. Fertility issues had plagued one of the women, Elizabeth Bordeaux, and her husband for three years. Pursuing adoption, they were completely staggered by the cost of the adoption process, which was at least $35,000 through a well-known adoption agency. The financial cost was daunting for a young married couple. What could they possibly do?

Elizabeth began to investigate the cost of private adoptions. Her detective work revealed much of the cost was devoted to advertising and personnel costs. Because of her experience as a media buyer for an advertising agency, she said to herself, "I can do that." In addition, she discovered the legal and certification costs were approximately $10,000. After praying for a time, she decided to market herself on social media in hopes of connecting with a birth mom. In a few months she did just that–connecting with a prospective birth mom. Soon she arranged the legal requirements herself, and she and her husband easily raised the $12,000 cost. At least it was easier than $35,000+. In a few more months they completed their low cost, self-marketed adoption plan for less than $12,000. Whoever heard of such a thing?

She shared the good news with Casey Brown, who also had struggled with fertility issues. Casey and her husband decided to try the same self-marketing technique, which they called "self-matching." They raised $7,500 and accomplished their adoption in less than 6 months as well. Then Casey and Elizabeth helped five of their friends, using the same marketing strategy, and all of them had their adoptions completed in less than six months and for less than $10,000 apiece. Elizabeth and Casey now believed they had found a better way.

After further prayer they decided to initiate a non-profit ministry called Quiver Full Adoptions in January 2017, giving up their ownership and for-profit status. The ministry helps birth moms connect with prospective adoptive parents as a licensed, child-placing agency. In the last eighteen months (2015-2016), Quiver Full Adoptions has completed thirty-five domestic adoptions legally with state certification for an average of $11,000 each. Most of these adoptions are completed in less than six months, far less than the national average of twenty-four months with traditional agencies.

Their clients, who become like family, are extremely pleased with the services they provide for birth mothers, which includes budget, marriage, and postpartum counseling. Surprisingly, most of their birth moms are married women whose motivation for placing their children for adoption is primarily financial considerations, which is the reason for the financial/budget counseling. Although told by multiple naysayers that their idea would never work, these two visionaries, Elizabeth and Casey, have found a better way and a "debt-free" way to help accomplish the adoption process. Someday I would not be surprised to hear they have franchised their concept to multiple other states.

"Bob! Bob! Wake up!"

"What? What's the matter?"

"I think we should invite Sarah to come live with us."

Bob sat straight up in bed. "Have you lost your mind? Are you crazy? What would we do with a sixteen-year old girl? I know who you are talking about; I've seen her at youth group. Trust me; that girl is no angel. How would she ever fit in to our family? She is completely different from us."

"I don't know. Maybe I am crazy! But would you at least just pray about it?"

It was 2:00 a.m. in the Smith's household, and thus began a journey of obedience to God that outsiders looking in would call foolish, but God looking down would bless immensely. Bob was a thirty-five-year old youth pastor at a church in South Carolina, while Barbara, his wife, taught English at a local high school. They had no children of their own due to medical reasons, but they considered all of the children in the youth group at church as their own. They loved and nurtured the kids in the youth group as if they belonged to them personally. Barbara often engaged in the lives of her school students who had personal and family issues in a way the average teacher did not. She connected with DSS workers trying to solve the issues confronting her students, for whom she cared deeply.

Then along came Sarah, a young sixteen-year old girl with long dark hair, dark eyes, and olive skin. She was captivatingly beautiful and an excellent student, but Barbara sensed deep and troubled waters underneath the surface. When Barbara first met her, Sarah had moved to her hometown with her stepmother and brother. She was new in Barbara's eleventh grade class when Barbara had to give her a tardy slip one morning. Later in the day Sarah returned to say, "Mrs. Smith, how can I undo this tardy slip? I can't afford to get into any more trouble. I am on probation." Immediately, Barbara's antennae went up. Most students didn't care one whit about a tardy slip; however, this girl was extremely upset.

Gradually, Barbara unraveled Sarah's tragic and complicated story. Her mother had died when she was six years of age. Her father remarried but then died of cancer when Sarah was twelve, leaving her in the hands of a stepmother–not a good situation. In fact, it was a terrible home situation. Her stepmother had multiple boyfriends. They constantly moved from town to town and school to school. She had been verbally, emotionally, and sexually abused at the hands of various family members over the years with no one to protect her. Her stepmother often physically assaulted her, pulling out handfuls of her long, beautiful hair. Sarah had to lie on top of her and hold her hands until her anger subsided.

Aware of this abuse, the extended family refused to do anything about it. After one particularly serious episode of physical abuse, Sarah took the family car, fleeing to another part of the state to hide out with other family and friends she thought might protect her. Vindictively, her stepmother filed charges against her for stealing the car. Some time later, when the juvenile court judge offered her detention time instead of returning home, Sarah chose time in the detention center. This response awakened her DSS worker to the severity of the abuse in her home.

Nevertheless, after the detention time she landed back home because she was still under age and had no other options. Her family then moved to the Smith's home town where the gracious hand of God began to move slowly in favor of this fallen angel as, unbeknownst to her, she was about to meet her earthly deliverers.

At this point, Sarah was finally removed from the home and placed in a children's home. Over the Christmas holidays this home transferred the children to a different facility in South Carolina. Previously, all of the orphans and foster children had been invited to Bob's church for youth events, so he had become acquainted with Sarah but only superficially. He knew who she was and could recognize her.

During the holidays, the news reported a teenage girl had run away from the children's home. It was Sarah. Bob said, "The entire two weeks of the holiday season, Barbara looked out the window to see if Sarah would walk up our drive. Every time the phone rang or the doorbell chimed she would jump, thinking it might be Sarah. Her heart was already attached to that little angel girl."

Sarah eventually returned to the children's home and then multiple foster homes. One Saturday morning her stepmom took her to a few yard sales then back to her home, where she began to pack up all of her personal belongings. Sarah asked her where she was going. The stepmom replied that she was returning to an old boyfriend, but when Sarah heard this, she knew she could not go to the home of a man who had previously sexually abused her.

On Monday morning Sarah sat in Barbara's classroom, crying uncontrollably. Barbara scooped her up, took her to the school office, and then said, "We're going home." Finding another teacher for her class, she did exactly that. Later, a DSS worker sat in the living room of Bob and Barbara Smith's home along with Sarah, discussing what it would take to have Sarah live with them.

God had prepared Bob with the aforementioned middle-of-the-night conversation when Barbara requested Bob to pray. God had also prepared Barbara with seeing Sarah's face day after day and hearing her heartbreaking story. In fact, God had been preparing them for just this moment for many years. Looking back, they realized that if they had had the children they lost to miscarriages, they might not have brought a troubled young woman into their home. In that moment, they understood some of the "whys" they had previously but briefly asked of God (like Job) in the years gone by. Although they had concluded they didn't have to know all the "whys" and just needed to live in the present and see what God is doing right now, they now understood more fully.

Bob looked at Sarah, who had been sitting quietly, and said, "Sarah, when God accepts us into His family, He takes us just as we are, no strings attached, but He doesn't expect us to stay as we are. He expects us to become like Him. I know this transition for you will be difficult; however, you need to ponder whether you really want to do this because we will have some guidelines in our home. I am a youth pastor and it doesn't look good for family members to smoke cigarettes. If you have to smoke, please smoke outside the house.

Furthermore, we are a church-going family, and you will be expected to go to church with the family." Sarah agreed to these household standards without hesitation.

Then Barbara made an amazing statement of acceptance and grace, especially considering Sarah was not their adopted child when she said, "This is your home. Everything we have is yours."

One week later, Sarah and Bob went to a gas station; oddly, she asked for chewing gum. "Why do you need gum?" he inquired.

"I just need something to chew on if I'm going to quit smoking," replied Sarah with a sheepish grin. She never smoked again.

Ever the pastor/teacher, Bob explained to my wife and me:

> We didn't know what we were going to get when we took Sarah into our home. Obviously, she had a turbulent background in her home of drugs, smoking, and profanity. She wore baggy britches and chains for jewelry; then she shaved off all of her long, beautiful dark hair except for two strands on either side of her face shortly after moving in with us. Talk about traumatic! Barbara's sister exclaimed, "What are you thinking? Are you out of your minds?"

> We wondered at times if we were out of our minds, but our love for Sarah was enough. We were willing to take the risk out of love for her and out of obedience to God's leadership in our lives. When something is right, you just know it and you just do it.

He continued with tears in his eyes.

> You know that's the way it is with our heav-
> enly Father. He takes us just the way we are
> with all of our baggage from our past, all of
> our sins and rebellion. He accepts us into
> His family, but He expects us to, over time,
> become like Him, to become conformed to
> the image of His Son. He expects us to put off
> the old man and "put on the new man, created
> to be like God in true righteousness and holi-
> ness," (Ephesians 4:24).

Of course, Sarah attended church with Bob and Barbara, but adopting their Christian belief was another thing. She watched them and their church family carefully for two years. The church family prayed for her diligently. Unconditional love flowed from the church body to Sarah so that she slowly began to become more and more like the Smith family and like the church family in her lifestyle and thinking. (Even her style of clothing changed from the baggy, black, Goth dress of her past.) Bob and Barbara anxiously waited for the moment of Sarah's salvation, but they understood it had to be in God's timing.

The biggest roadblock to salvation for Sarah was ques-tioning the goodness of God in allowing the troubles of her past. Bob encouraged her to consider the blessings of the present and not the unexplained questions of the past. Slowly, Sarah began to recognize God's care through the years and certainly in the present through Bob and Barbara as they cared for her as God the Father cares for us. From her own mouth she proclaimed, "I realized somebody cared and would not mistreat me, giving me an opportunity at life." Yes, they gave her an opportunity at life as God the Father gives us the opportunity for the abundant life and eternal life.

Finally, Sarah attended a church youth event attended by numerous youth and their leaders. Sensing the presence of the Holy Spirit at the end of the program, she stood up and looked for Bob. After conferring with him, together they walked to the front of the church for her to publicly confess Jesus Christ as her Lord and Savior. As they walked, Bob sent the thumbs up signal to his youth pastor friends, and a spontaneous celebration erupted — both in church and in heaven. This daughter had come home!

Two years later, Sarah announced she wanted to be a Smith. Despite now being an adult who could declare complete emancipation from adult authority in her life, she wanted to be fully adopted into Bob and Barbara's family, an arrangement they gladly and quickly made for this girl who had always been their daughter in their hearts.

Fifteen years later, as my wife and I made our way to the Smith's kitchen table, we passed by an absolutely gorgeous portrait of a lovely young bride. We were truly struck by her beauty. Their precious daughter married a man who had watched her story unfold in their church. She attended college on scholarships and now teaches school, where she watches for and helps students who show signs of similar life experiences. Best of all (we can say this because we are grandparents), the Smiths have two grandchildren of their very own, only made possible by their willingness to be submissive to God's call on their lives to bring home an angel with tarnished wings.

Sarah came to Bob and Barbara with a wretched past, including multiple foster homes, children's homes, physical and emotional abuse, and exposure to alcohol and drugs. Like Sarah, we come to the heavenly Father in much the same way. The "father of lies," (John 8:44) the Devil, has abused us in unimaginable ways. He leads us into temptation and sin designed to make us captives for a lifetime. Jesus emphatically asserted to the Pharisees that they "were of their father the devil," (John 8:44 NIV). This was no less true of you and me before being born again. Satan is a vindictive father armed with cruel hate. As the father of lies, he deceives and abuses his children in every way possible.

Nevertheless, in the fullness of time, along came our Deliverer. He wasn't a social worker. He wasn't a DSS representative. He wasn't the government! He was King Jesus, the Prince of Peace, the great Lion of Judah, the Savior of all mankind. He took hold of that incorrigible, abusive, lying king of terrors and loosed every blood-bought child of the King from his cold, tenacious grasp saying, "I am now his legal Advocate. You can't have him/her any longer. In fact, he/she is going to live in my Father's house!!"

Suddenly, we were adopted into the family of God, our names written down in the Lamb's Book of Life, and our feet set down on the Solid Rock. We were instantly transferred from the domain of darkness into the Kingdom of God's beloved Son. We were delivered from darkness into God's marvelous light. It's a glorious thing to be a child of the King! Then the Heavenly Father lovingly declared to you and me, "Child, look around; whatever is ours is yours. You've been adopted into my family."

Continuing to preach a little, Bob said, "God likes to take our mess and make a message. He took the mess of Sarah's life and made a great message of love and redemption.

> *"God likes to take our mess and make a message."*

We were all small players in this unfolding drama. Everybody around us watched intently, but Jesus was the Director and He gets all the glory!"

I don't know if it's because he shares his hunting adventures with me or because he's an all around nice guy, but Lee Lipford is one of my favorite people. His wife, Rebecca, is not just a lovely lady, but she also processes all of his deer meat for him. For all of us deer hunters, that's a huge plus in a wife. For their twenty-fifth wedding anniversary, he offered to take her anywhere she wanted to go. She said, "Let's go elk hunting. I want to know what's so exciting about elk hunting." So they drove out west and together, carrying all their gear, walked eight miles up into the mountains to his favorite hunting site and set up a base camp. How romantic!

After several days of hunting, Lee stood on a ridge overlooking the base camp, about 500 yards away, when he spied a herd of elk running in the direction of the camp with a large bull elk in the rear. He immediately dropped down, propped his rifle on a small tree, sited in, and took his best shot. The big bull staggered, so he knew it was a good shot.

He arrived in camp a little later to find Rebecca extremely excited. "You won't believe what just happened! A herd of elk charged toward camp, and I got it all on my camcorder and guess what?! Somebody up on the ridge took a shot at the bull and I got it on camera!"

"Oh, yeah!? Guess what?"

"What?"

"That somebody was me!"

After forty-five minutes of tracking the blood trail, they found the bull elk. The elk's rack missed the Boone and Crocket record book by only forty points. I admired the elk's shoulder mount in Lee's den when I visited their home. (Rebecca also cooks delicious venison barbecue, which I gratefully sampled the night I visited them.)

Lee and Rebecca are not just great outdoors people with interesting adventures. They are fine Christian people with spiritual depth that weathers the storms of life. Do you remember the parable that Jesus told about the man who built his house on the solid rock? "And when the storms came and beat upon his house it would not fall because it was built upon a strong foundation," (Matthew 7:24-27). Despite life not being kind to them, Lee and Rebecca have survived and prospered because, like the man in the parable, they built their lives upon a strong foundation.

THE LIPFORDS

One morning we heard a loud banging on the back door at 2 a.m. One of our nineteen-year old son's friends stood at the door, frantically crying and babbling, "Mr. Lee! Mr. Lee! Rusty's been in an accident and he's hurt real bad!"

"Who is that, Lee?" asked Rebecca.

"One of Rusty's friends."

"What does he want?"

"I don't know."

"Was he drunk?"

"I don't know. He says Rusty was in an accident."

"Lee, they don't send kids to inform parents that their children have been hurt in an accident."

"Yes, I know that's not proper, but get dressed; we need to go find out."

After we dressed and hurried to our car, we observed a police cruiser slowly turn down our street then put on his turn signal at our driveway. Rebecca said, "My knees got weak and I fell against the car. Immediately, the Scripture came to mind, 'No more pain, no more sorrow, no more tears.' I knew then that my son, Rusty, was with Jesus." He was gone.

Their grief was real; their sorrow was painful, but their house was built upon Jesus, the Rock of Ages.

THE LIPFORDS

"Do we have everything we need for the party?" asked Rebecca.

"Yes ma'am. We've got cake and hats and horns," said Lee.

Lee and Rebecca, now fifty-five years of age, were preparing for the one-year old birthday party of their grandson, also named Rusty. Their four-year old granddaughter Savannah was quite excited by all the preparation. They were waiting on Mark and Caroline, the parents of their grandchildren, who had been having some marital issues and were having some time alone to talk things out.

THE LIPFORDS

"What's keeping them? This ice cream cake won't keep forever."

"I don't know, Darling. I think I will go check on them."

Lee shared with me that on the way to see where they were, "God spoke to me in as clear a voice as you and I are talking today and said to me, 'Lee, don't worry. Caroline is with me now.' I called Rebecca and told her, 'Prepare yourself for the worst, but don't worry because Caroline is with Jesus.'"

They found out later that day both Mark and Caroline had been killed in a tragic accident. They had been married only five years with two precious little children, Rusty and Savannah.

THE LIPFORDS

Once again, we plunged into grief and sorrow. We felt like Job, like everything had been taken away from us, everything of real value. We would gladly give houses, cars, and land to have our children back again. We would gladly even give our own lives to give life to our children. You're not supposed to bury your children. Now not one, but two were gone; both of our children were gone. They were all we had. We were bereft — like Job.

We did not know how to curse God and die, as Job's wife suggested. It was just not in us to do so. Besides, we had two precious grandchildren who needed us. Life had to go on. We lost everything of real value, but God gave it back to us in these two grandchildren. It's funny because we prayed about adopting after Rusty died, but we never followed through with it; then these two children fell out of the sky and into our laps. In truth, these children were as much our salvation as we were theirs.

Taking these precious children into our house did not take any conscious decision. We just knew it was what God wanted us to do. We didn't have to think about taking them into our home; it was just the right thing to do, and it was what we wanted to do. We've never regretted it.

I asked Rebecca if she ever got mad at God in the beginning, "No, I didn't have time to be mad at God. I was too busy taking care of these two children. More than that, I can't afford to be mad at God."

Lee responded, "Yes, for a little while I was angry. I went to my favorite hunting spot, climbed the tallest oak tree, shook my fist at God, and screamed at Him for ten minutes until I got all my anger out. Then, I climbed down, got on my knees, and worshiped him like Job did. "

I looked at Lee and asked him, "Honestly, did you really do that?"

With humility he answered, "Yes, I really did. I'm not a perfect guy, but my house is built on the Rock."

24 Therefore everyone who hears these words of Mine and acts on them, may be compared to a wise man who built his house on the rock. 25 And the rain fell, and the floods came, and the winds blew and slammed against that house; and *yet* it did not fall, for it had been founded on the rock. 26 Everyone who hears these words of Mine and does not act on them, will be like a foolish man who built his house on the sand. 27 The rain fell, and the floods came, and the winds blew and slammed against that house; and it fell—and great was its fall. Matthew 7:24-27

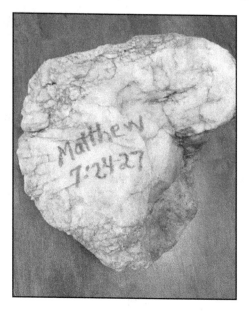

The rock in the Lipford's home

RESOURCE (for adoption services)
Bethany Christian Services
901 Eastern Avenue, NE
Grand Rapids, Michigan 49503
800.238.4269
www.bethany.org

Quiver Full Adoptions, Inc.
QuiverFullAdoptions@gmail.com
412-C Pettigru Street
Greenville, SC 29601
864.334.8593

Chapter Sixteen

Uncle Jim's Folly

J ane, an attractive college student pursuing a degree at a
local university in health sciences, sat on my exam table
staring at the wall with anger in her eyes. "My whole family
is divided because of me! I don't know what to do. Half of
them want me to go to court and testify. If I do, the other half
will hate me and never speak to me again."

Totally bewildered, I had no idea what she was talking
about. I held up both hands with palms up, shrugged my
shoulders, and looked at her. I waited patiently while she
stared at me with those angry eyes. Suddenly, she began to
cry uncontrollably, putting her hands to her face. I put my
arms around her shoulders and stood still for several minutes
while she composed herself.

"Dr. Jackson, after my dad left us, Uncle Jim began to
visit us often. We thought he was our protector. I was just an
elementary school girl when he first came around. I looked
up to him. He took me places and bought me ice cream and
Christmas presents. He did nice things for Mom around the
house." She started to weep silently a few moments, but then
the anger returned to her voice. "When I was thirteen, he
came around when Mom was not home and played games
with me, sexual games, and told me not to tell my mom. Dr.
Jackson, he molested me, but I was afraid he would never
come back to help my mom, so I just kept quiet. For years,
I kept quiet.

"When I became an older teenager, he brought me nice gifts and nice clothes. The molestation became more invasive and more aggressive. He played mind games with me. He told me it was really all my fault, that I had tempted him and seduced him. I was so confused because he was an adult, an authority figure my mom trusted. When he left me, he always warned me not to let my mom find out because she would be so disappointed in me. He not only abused me sexually, but he manipulated me mentally." Jane stopped and took several deep breaths.

I was shocked by this revelation. I knew her uncle well. He was a prominent businessman in our city and active in a local church. I know that the "heart of man is deceitful and desperately wicked," but I am astounded at the continual revelations of that wickedness, especially in so-called Christian people.

She then looked at me with a vacant expression and spoke with a far away voice, "When I was sixteen, I became pregnant. At first I was just afraid, then I realized I had a way out of this torment. I had a way to expose Uncle Jim and escape from him. Suddenly, I became happy. Really, I was exhilarated. I kept it from Uncle Jim and my mother for four and a half months. Finally, my mother figured it out. Of course, she accused me of messing around with one of my male friends at school. Thinking that I would find freedom, I triumphantly exposed Uncle Jim. My mother slapped me and called me a liar and a tramp. I can't tell you how devastated I was that she would not believe me. We said nothing to each other for two days.

"Two days later, Uncle Jim came for a visit. As usual, he brought presents. He was all happy when he came in. In my desperation, I lifted my shirt and said, 'Look what you've done to me.' The look on his face gave him away. Immediately, my mother began to attack him, screaming at him. He denied it all, but I had secret cell phone photos of him getting dressed in my bathroom that he did not know about. When I brought them out, he crumbled and confessed."

Jane then began to weep silently and trembled all over. "Dr. Jackson, things didn't go as I thought they would. The baby was supposed to be my salvation, my way out of this sordid, six-year ordeal. Oh, but no, my mom and Uncle Jim had long discussions behind my back. They both showed up one day and said we were going on a trip to Atlanta. I didn't want to go anywhere with Uncle Jim, but my mom persuaded me. We rode in silence, nobody speaking, until we arrived at an abortion clinic. I was so stunned I couldn't speak. They told me it was the best thing for the family, and before I knew it the procedure was done and we were driving home. I no longer had a baby. I was so shocked I couldn't even cry. Uncle Jim whistled all the way home."

Suddenly, it made sense to me why she had been in and out of my office for the last few years for panic attacks and depression. My heart was broken for this attractive college girl. I had known nothing about any of this trauma in her life. She continued, "My mother has slowly come over to my side. We have attended counseling together. We have decided to bring charges against Uncle Jim. He has denied them outright. Half the family believes us; half the family believes him. It has completely divided our family. You wouldn't believe what some of my family has said about my Mom and me. I have to appear in court next week, but I am terrified to face Uncle Jim. I can't concentrate on my schoolwork; I can't sleep and I cry all the time."

Secret sins eat away at the fabric of families for generations. Yet lies, deceit, and immorality must be exposed to the light of day or healing can never occur. "Have nothing to do with the fruitless deeds of darkness, but rather expose them. For it is shameful even to mention what the disobedient do in secret. But everything exposed by the light becomes visible, for it is light that makes everything visible," (Eph. 5:11-14 NIV).

Now I know what many people will think after reading Jane's story. "Well, shoot dog! That abortion really was the best thing for that girl and that family. That girl didn't want to raise a child conceived from incest. Neither did that family." Well, let's look at the actual research.

It is commonly assumed that women who become pregnant as a result of rape or incest would want an abortion to put the "assault behind them, recover more quickly, and avoid the additional trauma of giving birth to a rapist's child," or the child of an incestuous relation but, in fact, an early study in 1979 by Dr. Sandra Mahkorn showed that 75-85% of rape victims who conceived did not obtain abortions.[1] From a sample of 164 pregnant rape victims, Dr. David C. Reardon reports a similar number of 73% in an article in 1993.[2] This should cause us to pause and reconsider our perception that abortion is wanted or even best for rape victims.

Why would these women not choose abortion? Answering this question is an important book called *Victims and Victors: Speaking Out About their Pregnancies, Abortions and Children Resulting from Sexual Assault*, which is based on the largest survey of sexually assaulted women who became pregnant.[3] One of the authors, Dr. Reardon, summarizes why most women who become pregnant as a result of sexual assault do not want to abort.

> Many women who become pregnant through sexual assault do not believe in abortion, believing it would be a further act of violence perpetrated against their bodies and their children. Further, many believe that their children's lives may have some intrinsic meaning or purpose which they do not yet understand. This child was brought into their lives by a

horrible, repulsive act. But perhaps God (or fate as some would say), will use the child for some greater purpose. Good can come from evil. The woman may also sense, at least at a subconscious level, that if she can get through the pregnancy she will have conquered the rape. By giving birth, she can reclaim some of her lost self-esteem. Giving birth, especially when conception was not desired, is a totally selfless act, a generous act, a display of courage, strength, and honor. It is proof that she is better than the rapist. While he was selfish, she can be generous. While he destroyed, she can nurture.[4]

For those who did abort, Reardon states they felt pressured by family members or health care workers to have abortions even when the women did not want an abortion.[5] Usually, in the case of incest and sometimes over the girl's objections, the girl's parents or the perpetrator make the decision and arrangements for the abortion, not the girl herself, and in a few cases, the victim was not even clearly aware that she was pregnant or that the abortion was being carried out.[6]

Dr. George Maloof, in his article "The Consequences of Incest: Giving and Taking Life," says incest victims rarely ever voluntarily agree to abortion; plus, when covered up, the incestuous behavior can be passed from one generation to another.[7] Reardon contends that "the incest victim is more likely to see the pregnancy as a way out of the incestuous relationship because the birth of her child will expose the sexual activity. She is also likely to see in her pregnancy the hope of bearing a child with whom she can establish a truly loving relationship, one far different than the exploitative relationship in which she has been trapped."[8] This is exactly what my patient Jane thought.

Last, but not least, we must listen to those who were conceived as a result of rape. Remembering her mother's courage and selflessness, Rebecca Wasser-Kiessling, who was conceived as a result of rape, "reminds us of a fundamental truth that transcends biological paternity: 'I believe that God rewarded my birth mother for the suffering she endured, and that I am a gift to her. The serial rapist is not my creator; God is.'"[9] Another woman conceived during a rape, Julie Makimaa, proclaims, "It doesn't matter how I began. What matters is who I will become."[10]

After all, it is a twisted logic that would kill the unborn child for the misdeed of one of the parents.

After all, it is a twisted logic that would kill the unborn child for the misdeed of one of the parents. In America, we do not execute the child for the crimes of the parent. That only happens in third world countries ruled by cruel dictators.

I continue to see Jane routinely for other medical issues unrelated to her pathological family relationship. Eventually, she testified against her Uncle Jim. He was convicted and sentenced to a long term in prison. The nail in his coffin was the check that he used to pay for her abortion, proving the truthfulness of her story. Half the family rejoiced; half the family grieved. The scripture says, "...be sure your sin will find you out," (Numbers 32:23). Uncle Jim was a churchgoing man. He should have known that.

Jane's personal healing process was long and difficult. She eventually married and graduated from nursing school. The last time I saw her she was about eight months pregnant, radiantly beautiful, and glowing like a pregnant woman should.

Chapter Seventeen

Save Yourself

The principal's voice came over the PA system at the local high school, "Good morning, Students! Class will be dismissed after lunch today for Thanksgiving holidays. All of you taking the SAT exam Saturday must be present by 7:45 a.m. Bring two freshly sharpened #2 pencils and a personal ID. If you continue to use illicit, injectable drugs, you should stop by the nurse's office on your way home and pick up sterile needles and syringes. Have a safe and happy holiday."

This was the beginning of a presentation I made to 400 students at a large high school in my home county. The students were the elected student government representatives from every high school in our county. I had been asked to debate a doctor's wife about the merits of abstinence education, which had been mandated by law in our state. The students sat in stunned silence as I discussed the folly of offering sterile needles to drug abusers through a school nurse and how that would only encourage more of the unsafe and illicit drug abuse. More than that, it would be illegal.

I then began to make the comparison to the school programs cropping up nationwide offering birth control devices to high school students without parental knowledge. My contention was that it would encourage more of the undesired behavior. It was immoral, and it undermined parental authority. The longer I talked, the more restless the students became. When I began to speak about immoral behavior and cutting parents out of the loop, they began to jeer me openly, hooting and trying to shout me down. The school officials merely shrugged as if they were helpless. My female opponent in the debate was received politely, since her contention was that teen sexual activity was inevitable so free birth control should be given by schools to protect students. During the question and answer time afterwards, she received no questions at all. However, I received a barrage of questions. I couldn't even answer them all. They were not polite in the least. The students' questions were angry and challenging. God gave me grace and enabled me to keep my composure. Thankfully, I was prepared and I knew my perspective well.

One student even asked me if I was a virgin when I got married. I laughed, "I had plenty of opportunities to lose my virginity just like my classmates in school and just like you. However, I'll tell you what I told my friends growing up–I can become a fornicator like you any time I want to, but you can never become a virgin like me ever again. You've given the best fruit out of the garden of your life to someone else who may not be your husband or wife, and you can't get it back. You'll never be able to look at your bride or groom on your wedding day and say, 'Baby, I saved myself just for you,' but I can."

A deathly silence fell over the student body. A few boyfriends and girlfriends looked at each other. The students on the front row, who obviously supported me, smiled broadly in appreciation. The rest sat totally bumfuzzled. Then one student shouted, "That's not even possible." The whole room erupted into confusion once again. God help us! Those were the future leaders in America!

Afterwards, a few students and teachers came up to me and apologized for the behavior of the entire group. One of the most vocal hecklers, a young black male student, came up to me and told me he disagreed with me strongly but respected me for not losing my composure. It was an emotionally exhausting experience to be shouted down by 400 students. What left me dismayed was that these were supposed to be the best students in each of our county's schools. Again, these were the elected student government representatives from every high school in our county. Did this represent the moral milieu in which our students went to school?

I include this anecdote (and this chapter) because early in my prolife journey I spent a great deal of time speaking in churches, schools, and public forums promoting the merits of abstinence education. As we all intuitively know, young people who respect one another and choose to save themselves until marriage tend not to experience unwanted pregnancies nor do they seek out abortion services. Promoting moral integrity and abstinence until marriage is the biblical standard. I recognize that this is foolishness to the lost world – hence, the heckling from 400 students. It definitely requires the grace of God and the indwelling power of the Holy Spirit for high school and college students to save themselves until marriage. As God-fearing and right-thinking adults, we should always encourage and support our young people to walk in the light and to live by God's principles of life. God's ways are always the best ways. Galatians 6:8 says, "For the one who sows to his own flesh shall from the flesh reap corruption, but the one who sows to the Spirit shall from the Spirit reap eternal life."

In the late 1980s, my medical partner and I were the first doctors in the county to affiliate with a statewide HMO sponsored by a major medical insurer in South Carolina. It was a financial boon to our medical practice. We inherited several large industries in our county that also signed up with the HMO. Many of these patients who came with that decision are still my patients today, and we are best of friends. Additionally, the school district signed up with the HMO, and we received a large influx of schoolteachers and school administrators as new patients.

As many of you know, one of the commitments of an HMO that helps it conserve money is it requires the family doctor, the gatekeeper, to provide all of the services he is trained to do rather than refer to a specialist, who usually provides the same services at a higher cost. That didn't sit well with many patients who thought we would just refer them to the specialist whom they had always seen, which we did if they had serious medical issues. If they did not, we were required to care for those patients ourselves. This especially did not please women who were attached to their gynecological doctors.

To make matters worse, my partners and I had always had a policy that we did not prescribe birth control to unmarried women unless they planned to marry within a few months or unless they had a menstrual disorder. (Now don't get in a fizz; I don't prescribe medicines like Viagra to unmarried men, either.) Why would we not do that when it is so culturally acceptable in the medical community? We have a strong conviction that prescribing birth control to unmarried women would allow them to pursue a lifestyle physically dangerous and unhealthy, plus spiritually and emotionally devastating. Sexual activity outside of marriage (promiscuity) often leads to a multitude of sexually transmitted diseases, which I am compelled to treat all too many times. These are entirely preventable if my patients would just save themselves until marriage.

Abstinence until marriage protects my patients from the numerous sexually transmitted diseases that abound. That is not impossible, as so many people believe. Our young people are not unable to control themselves. Please give them some credit and don't give them sterile needles–I mean–drug paraphernalia (birth control pills) that enables them to pursue their permissive lifestyles without consequences. The only problem is there *are* consequences; they don't use their birth control properly and they still contract STDs. They still get pregnant before marriage. They still get broken hearts.

———— · ▬ ··◆··· ▬ · ————

Betsy was a twenty-four-year old telemarketer who complained of sores on her private parts. Upon an examination, she was found to have genital herpes. I informed her of the diagnosis, whereupon she began to cry a bucket of tears. When she finally composed herself, she cried out loud, "How could this happen to me?"

I knew the answer was obvious and the question rhetorical, but I felt compelled to point out the obvious. I reminded her of our conversation a year ago when I warned her that her premarital sexual activity would result in her getting "burned" just as Proverbs 6:27 says. Once again I repeated that verse– "Can a man take fire in his bosom and not get burned?" She hung her head in shame and began to weep once again. She admitted, "Dr. Jackson, you are so right. I should have listened to you. This won't ever go away, will it?"

"No, ma'am. It won't." Again, the tears flowed. We had a long discussion regarding the proper treatment of genital herpes and the merits of abstinence until marriage. She seemed ready to make that commitment now, but too late to avoid the long-term consequences of genital herpes. We family doctors have these conversations way too often, and it breaks my heart. An ounce of abstinence would prevent a pound of heartache. Now she would have to tell her eventual fiancé/husband that she has herpes before she could marry him. I'm reminded of Moses' warning to the Israelites before they entered the Promised Lands when he said, "Be sure that your sins will find you out," (Numbers 32:23).

Andre sat on the exam table in Room #2 complaining of urethral drainage for one week. His on again/off again girlfriend had been diagnosed with an STD. I had already treated him for an STD once before and had strongly advised him to save himself until marriage. At that encounter he had laughed up his sleeve at me. Now he was back with the same complaint, sheepish and embarrassed. We obtained appropriate lab tests and prescribed an antibiotic. I then asked him, "Do you plan to marry this girl?"

"Oh no, we fuss and fight too much."

"Then why are you sexually involved with a girl that you do not intend to marry?"

He was startled and confused by that question. "I don't know, sir."

"Don't you think you should make up your mind about the future of your relationship before you continue to engage in sexual relations? You know that you become one flesh with the person with whom you have sexual intimacy. If you don't plan to marry her and you don't get along very well, you should not get involved sexually."

He looked at the floor for a while, then said, "I know you are right. It's just so hard."

"Look, Andre. This isn't how your mama raised you. It is hard to go back to holding hands once you have been intimate, but you've got to man up and be the leader in the relationship. Either marry this girl and be a man of integrity or break it off and save yourself for the right girl in your life. That way you won't keep getting these infections, and you'll have a clear conscience before God."

I continued, "By the way, how's your prayer life? Are you still going to church with your mama?" He just stared at his shoes. "That's what I thought. It's hard to talk to God when you've been screwing around." He just nodded. "Andre, sex outside of marriage will always wreck your spiritual life. It drives a wedge between you and God. You don't want to live like this the rest of your life. You need to confess, repent, and make things right with God and your girlfriend. I'm not against you, Andre; I'm for you. I want you to be healthy– physically and spiritually."

"I know what you mean, and I know you are right," Andre replied. I knew his parents well. His mother was a godly woman who had tried to raise him right. Sadly, I had treated his dad for an STD three different times, which was why his parents were separated. Deuteronomy 5:9 says, "...I, the Lord your God, am a jealous God, visiting the iniquity of the fathers on the children, and on the third and the fourth generations of those who hate Me." (I was hopeful his mother's influence would help him break the cycle.)

Oddly enough, as soon as I left Andre, I walked into Exam Room #3 and encountered Philip, whose wife had abandoned him for another man several years previously. He had plunged into a deep depression for about two years. He lost a lot of weight and was barely functional at work. He required antidepressant medication and intensive counseling. Now about six years later he had met another woman and was in to see me for counseling. The issue of the day was the new woman had herpes. He was inquiring about medication to protect himself from acquiring this viral infection.

"Well, congratulations. When do you plan to get married?" That was always my introductory question to set the stage for further discussion.

"We're not sure yet that we are going to get married," he replied.

"Well, shoot dog. Phillip, aren't you putting the cart before the horse? You don't need a medication to protect you from herpes; you need something to protect you from intercourse. You are a Christian man. You know good and well you shouldn't be sexually involved before you marry!"

His eyes, which always bugged out a little bit, just about popped out of his head. He just stared speechless for several minutes. I sat quietly, allowing the Holy Spirit to do His job. Then Phillip dropped his head and stared at the floor. His shoulders heaved and tears began to flow. "I know, Dr. Jackson, but it's just so hard."

"Look, Phillip, you know when you become sexually intimate you become one flesh with your girlfriend, and you will never again be able to separate yourself from her emotionally or physically or spiritually. That's the way it was with your wife, wasn't it?" He shook all over and nodded affirmatively.

"If you become one flesh with her before marriage, you will never be able to hear the subtle prompting of Holy Spirit. All you will hear is the bass drum of your hormones pounding in your ears. You won't be able to make logical decisions. You will only make emotional decisions. In fact, that is probably where you are now, or you would not be thinking about committing adultery with a woman who has herpes. That's not very intelligent or Christian!"

He nodded once again and really began to sob. "Phillip, I'm not against you, brother; I'm for you. More than that, how can you ask me to give you a medication that would make me complicit in helping you commit adultery and perhaps acquiring an infection you would never be rid of? I can't in good conscience do that. If I am your really good friend, I would warn you of the dangerous path you are traveling on."

"There is a way which seems right to a man, but its end is the way of death," (Proverbs 14:12).

We both sat silently for several minutes. Then he looked up at me, wiped the tears away, and with a white blanched face, said, "Thanks, Doc, I needed to hear that. I was about to make a terrible mistake. I know God brought me here today just to hear you say that." He then threw his arms around my neck, gave me a bear hug, and slowly walked away with stooped shoulders. "A rebuke goes deeper into one who has understanding than a hundred blows into a fool," (Proverbs 17:10). Speaking the truth in love — sometimes you win and sometimes you lose.

———————— · ▬ ··◆·· ▬ · ————————

Now back to the schoolteachers that the HMO brought to our medical office. We collected a large number of unmarried, female schoolteachers who were accustomed to going to OB-GYN doctors annually for birth control devices to prevent pregnancy, no questions asked. Well, we were not those doctors. The conversations followed two main tracks.

"Doctor, by the way, I need a refill for my birth control pills."

"Are you married?"

"No."

"Do you plan to be married in the next six months?"

"No."

"You just told me your cycle was regular. Right?"

"Yes."

"So I conclude you need birth control to prevent pregnancy. Correct?"

"Yes."

"Let's have a little conversation about this. Our office policy is not to prescribe birth control to unmarried women merely to prevent pregnancy. We believe that it allows you to pursue a lifestyle that is physically unhealthy and spiritually/emotionally devastating. We cannot in good conscious facilitate that lifestyle. Birth control devices don't protect you from sexually transmitted diseases nor from a broken heart when your boyfriend takes the best fruit out of your garden then decides to leave you, used and abused. Has that already happened to you? (Often the answer was an embarrassed "yes.") Birth control won't protect your tender heart!

More than that, they aren't 100% effective. Are you ready to be pregnant?"

A horrified look often came over their face.

"No, I didn't think so. Again birth control devices don't always protect one from pregnancy. Most importantly, they don't protect you from the impact on your spiritual life. Illicit sex will drive you away from God. Can you still pray or go to church? How can I in good conscience prescribe a medication that will harm you in all of these areas?"

Response #1 — About 50% of our young female patients listened politely, but fumed inside. They were stiff and rigid on the outside with their eyes glazed over. Some were flushed with shame and embarrassment that someone would have the gall to call them out on their sinful, dangerous lifestyle, but they still would not receive my advice to save themselves until marriage.

About 20% would be livid with rage, getting red in the face and rejecting every common sense word of advice that I had uttered. Some of these really mad young ladies told me off in no uncertain terms. I got used to it, but it greatly saddened my heart. Remember, back then I was about the same age as many of these young schoolteachers. Usually, they would not curse me, but they did curse my employees on their way out the door after not paying for services rendered since the physical exam wasn't what they were really interested in, just the birth control.

Often I gave them a three-month supply of birth control pills, asked them to think over my advice, and reminded them they could easily obtain birth control at the health department if that was the lifestyle they really wanted to pursue. I gave them the three-month supply because we were both in a difficult position. The HMO forced these women to come to our office for health care, and we had not had a chance to develop a patient/doctor relationship with an understanding of our office policies. I was in a difficult position of violating my conscience and our office policy merely to accommodate an influx of intelligent, attractive, well-paying patients who obviously would not share the philosophy of our medical practice over the long haul.

If we were to compromise our convictions, it would have been a great practice builder to keep all of these young teachers who would have eventually married, had babies, and brought their children to our practice. We chose, rather, to speak the truth in love and let the chips fall where they may. All of these women had now had at least one person to lovingly and respectfully speak the truth into their lives regarding their immoral and irresponsible lifestyles. I never saw most of those women ever again, but I suspect they will never forget the doctor that confronted them with the truth regarding their illicit sexual lifestyle. I know I won't forget. It was emotionally exhausting for me.

Response #2 — About 30% listened carefully to my advice, looked at me sadly, and replied, "Dr. Jackson, you are right. I know you are right. My boyfriend and I have talked about this, but we just can't seem to stop. It is just like we are addicted to sex. We are both so ashamed. I would die if my parents found out we were involved sexually. You are exactly right about my spiritual life, too. I can't pray or read my Bible; I feel so guilty all the time. I haven't been to church in months."

At this point the young woman cried real tears of repentance. This happened so often I knew what she would say next. "Dr. Jackson, I just needed someone to tell me what to do." We would then have a conversation regarding the steps she needed to take to break free from this immoral lifestyle. Of course, I did not prescribe any birth control devices for this young lady. "He whose ear listens to the life-giving reproof will dwell among the wise," (Proverbs 15:31).

Many of my patients, young and old, live in sexual sin; fornication is the biblical term. They have a guilty conscience before God. All they need is a Christian friend they respect to call them out on it in a kind and respectful way. I don't just speak truth to young people. I have plenty of patients who live together for years and never marry–so-called common law marriages. I frequently challenge both male and female partners, asking them why they don't marry.

"'Johnny, how long have you and Brenda been living together?"

"Seven years."

"When are you going to marry her and create for her a secure relationship?"

"What do you mean?"

"Johnny, marriage is a sacred institution, designed by God in the very beginning to portray the mystical union between Jesus and His bride, the church. Marriage has cosmic and spiritual implications. Every divorce is a lie. It implies that Jesus would divorce His bride, the church, which we know would never happen. He said, 'Never will I leave you; never will I forsake you,' (Hebrews 13:5 NIV). If marriage is a picture of Jesus' union with His bride the church, what do you think living with a woman without marrying her says to the world?"

He looked at me quite confused. "I never thought about it."

"It presents a picture of Jesus as an adulterer like you."

Sweat beaded up on his forehead. He wiped it with the back of his hand. "Are you serious?"

"I'm dead serious. Is that the picture you and Brenda want to paint? Are you planning on leaving Brenda?"

"Well, no. We are stuck together like white on rice."

"What keeps you from getting married? Are you scared?"

"I ain't scared of nothing."

"Then I dee-double-dog dare you to ask her to marry you. Before I see you at the next six month visit, you better be married to that girl."

He looked confused again as he walked out of the exam room. However, when I saw Johnny six months later, he proudly showed me a wedding band, and brought Brenda with him to that visit. Honest, married people, they both wore proud smiles. I wish I could say many of my similar patients took up my challenge but that wouldn't be true. However, enough have, so I keep giving them the challenge. Sometimes folks just need an encouraging word, someone to speak the truth in love.

———— · —··•··— · ————

Rembert was disabled in a work related accident. He also had severe osteoarthritis and suffered significant joint pain in multiple joints all the time. When I first met him, he smoked like a freight train, drank booze like a fish, and cheated on his wife constantly. He drove a big Cadillac and dressed like a pimp. We were as different as night and day, but we got along famously despite the fact that every time I saw him, I dogged him to quit smoking, drinking, and carousing. After one of my mini-sermons, he asked, "Doctor, is that your best advice?"

"Yes, sir, it is."

"Well, how much would you charge me for your second best advice?" He was never serious with me. He developed emphysema at an early age, alcohol-related liver disease, and, as you might expect, his wife left him. Sounds like a country/western song, doesn't it? He was a miserable little man. He once told me I was his only friend in the whole world. I treated him respectfully, but I also told him the truth regarding the consequences of his dissolute lifestyle, all of which eventually came true. I also told him drunkards could not inherit the kingdom of God and that he would most certainly spend eternity in hell if he did not repent and believe on the name of Jesus as His only Savior. We had that conversation multiple times over the years.

Eventually, his wife (from whom he was divorced) died of heart failure due to uncontrolled hypertension. That threw him into a depression because he blamed himself for her early demise.

Then one day he showed up in my office with a great, big toothless smile on his face. "Dr. Jackson, I wanted you to be the first to know I got saved last Sunday."

"Rembert, are you for real?" Understandably, I was skeptical. He had lived a hard, immoral lifestyle. My patients often played the religion card to get on my good side before asking for narcotic drugs from my Christian partners and me.

"Yes, Dr. Jackson. I'm sho' 'nough for real. I've been going to this little church downtown and the Spirit of God got all over me Sunday, and I gave my life to the Lord. I'm a new man now." He continued to smile broadly.

I leaned over and gave him a big, rejoicing hug and asked, "What's next?"

"No more drinking booze for me," he exclaimed.

"Are you going to keep going to church?"

"Oh, yeah, me and Pastor John are the best of friends."

We talked a little bit about what it takes to grow and prosper as a new believer. He took it all in excitedly, and then he left praising God. I said to myself, "We'll see how long this lasts."

But it did last. Rembert was a new man in Christ. Miraculously, he quit drinking alcohol immediately, despite being an alcoholic for more than thirty years. He quit bugging me for narcotic pain relievers at every visit, further evidence that he was a changed man. He tried mightily to quit smoking, moving from two packs a day to half a pack a day (but he never fully quit).

Rembert became a faithful volunteer at the little church downtown, and eventually became a Sunday School teacher of young boys. I was really proud of how he progressed and stayed faithful to his commitment to Christ. Eventually, he met a young lady (twenty years younger than him) and they became an item.

One day he came to the office for routine meds for his arthritis and hypertension. As he was leaving, he brazenly asked if I had any samples of those blue pills. "You mean Viagra?" I asked.

"Yeah, doc, Viagra."

"Hold on, Rembert, what do you need Viagra for?"

"Doc, you know. My nature don't work so good anymore."

"I realize that, Rembert, but you are a Christian man now and you are not married. Have you been married since I last saw you?"

Whining, he said, "No, doc, I haven't."

"Well, Rembert, there is a disconnect here between your Christian faith and your lifestyle. Why would you want me to give you a medication that will help you do something immoral and contrary to your Christian conviction and mine? You are putting me in a bad spot."

"I haven't thought about that," he said, somewhat perplexed.

"Are you planning on marrying this girl?"

"No, not really."

"Rembert, the Bible calls that adultery." He began to squirm. "Are you ready to have that on your conscience?" No answer but more squirming. "Have you told Pastor John about your plans to commit adultery with one of his parishioners?" No answer. "I think you need to pray about this a little more. If you can get God's permission, then I'll change my mind." Rembert and I were at a variance on this issue. At every subsequent visit he would ask for Viagra, and I would decline.

It was one thing to have this conversation with Rembert, a previous alcoholic and philanderer. It was another thing to have this same conversation with deacons and elders after their wives had died. Believe me, I have had this same contest/conversation many times. These churchmen will meet a lady friend, often someone in their congregation or in another church, and they may or may not be contemplating marriage, but just as brazenly as Rembert, they ask me for a Viagra-type medicine to assist their sexual performance.

"Well, congratulations, brother. When do you plan to get married?" Immediately, my deacon/elder friend begins to squirm a bit.

"Oh, we're not planning to be married," my patient says. I stare at my deacon/elder/Christian brother and let the silence hang heavily in the room, allowing the Holy Spirit to work on their hearts for a few moments. "We know we shouldn't be intimate, but we just want to try things out before we make a full commitment to each other."

"My brother, you sound like twenty-year olds who cohabitate to see if they are compatible before they marry. You've condemned that all of your life. Are you really asking me to help you become an adulterer after you've served God faithfully all of these years in your church?" At this point these godly men will often become contrite, embarrassed, and thank me for keeping them from making a huge mistake in their spiritual lives. They become even stronger friends and faithful, loyal patients, thanking me repeatedly for speaking the truth to them in love. "My brethren, if any among you strays from the truth, and one turns him back, let him know that he who turns a sinner from the error of his way will save his soul from death, and will cover a multitude of sins," (James 5:19-20).

Sadly, some of these men become red in the face, angry, and defiant. Then they ask me who I think I am judging them. One particular gentleman, if I can call him that, was a retired public school administrator. Interestingly, like Rembert, his wife had died of heart failure about ten years prior. He was an elder in an Episcopal church when he requested medical assistance for his sexual life. I knew he wasn't married. I was taken aback that this seventy-year old man, who was prominent in the community and in his church, would consider extramarital sexual activity. After declining to assist him and giving him my rationale, he responded indignantly with a loud, angry voice, "I can't believe you would judge me like that." He was a big man and fifteen years older than me. I could tell he was accustomed to getting his way.

"My brother, only Jesus is the righteous Judge. I can judge no one. Nevertheless, I am instructed to be a fruit inspector. Jesus said, 'A good tree cannot produce bad fruit, nor can a bad tree produce good fruit... So then, you will know them by their fruits,' (Matthew 7:18-20). It doesn't seem to me any of your intentions will bring forth any fruit pleasing to the Lord. I have an obligation before God to warn you. 'Food gained by fraud tastes sweet to a man, but he ends up with a mouth full of gravel,' (Proverbs 20:17 NIV)."

At this he stared at me a long moment, jaw muscles clinching, his face red as a beet. Then he suddenly relaxed, slumped his shoulders, and walked out of my office without paying his bill. He had been my patient for twenty-plus years. I had cared for his wife for fifteen years, and his four daughters. He returned to see me in a few months, and we continued to be friends. He never mentioned that encounter. I heard through the grapevine he had broken off with his girlfriend. Speaking the truth is a little hard and a little dangerous to long-time relationships. You win some, and you lose some. "But speaking the truth in love, we are to grow up in all aspects into Him, who is the head, even Christ," (Ephesians 4:15).

Chapter Eighteen

Don't You Know Where Children Come From?

After our third child Miriam was born, people began to ask us the inevitable question, "Are you going to have any more children?" We were way over the national average of 1.87 children per family.[1] (I've never seen any of those 0.87 children, but I bet they are interesting). At that point we had not really given it much thought, since we both came from families with four children. We just thought we would have four children; like begets like.

This question eventually caused us to ponder exactly how many children we would have. Being Bible-believing Christians (are there any other kind?), we started looking into the scriptures to see what the Bible had to say about childbearing. We also asked other Christian people. We already had a pretty good idea about what the culture around us thought about children. Two children was the perfect family — me and mama, Beth and Bob, us four, and no more.

As a family doctor I saw a constant stream of young moms and dads who had two children coming to see me asking for a vasectomy or a tubal ligation to prevent further childbearing. I always felt obliged to point out to them that this was a permanent arrangement and that one of their children could possibly die of disease or accident. This rarely would dissuade the young parents. As I grew older, I asked them why they opposed having more children. Except for those who had previous c-sections, the answers were eerily the same. "We can't afford more than two children."

"We can't afford to send more than two to college."

"We can't handle more than two."

"How will we ever pay for the weddings?"

You get the drift. It was a financial calculation. Now most of my patient population lives in the suburbs and are fairly affluent. Usually both husband and wife work, although not always. Often, I was talking to two young professionals who both worked, who both drove fancy cars, and lived in a sizable home in an upscale neighborhood. They wouldn't admit it to me, but their primary concern would be that more children might cause them to have to scale down their standard of living. They loved their stuff more than children.

When I listened to my patients and to my friends with whom I had similar conversations, my mind often drifted to my father's family. My dad was the youngest of ten children, eight boys and two girls. His mother died a few months after he was born, so he and his three immediately older brothers were raised by his sixteen year-old sister, my Aunt Eunice. My grandfather Jackson worked for the Black River Co-op, an electric company, and farmed on the side to feed the family. As my uncles used to say, they were dirt farmers and they were dirt poor, but they loved each other and were generally happy. No food stamps or government programs existed back then. It was "root hog or die" every day.

My grandparents weren't concerned about paying for college or weddings or whether they could handle a bunch of kids. To them children were not a liability but a blessing, and they gladly received as many children as God would give them, as did many of their neighbors and friends. The Psalmist says, "Behold, children are a gift of the Lord; the fruit of the womb is a reward. Like arrows in the hand of a warrior, so are the children of one's youth. How blessed is the man whose quiver is full of them; they shall not be ashamed, when they speak with their enemies in the gate," (Psalm 127:3-5).

My grandparents believed that and practiced that. Their quiver was full and my grandfather was not put to shame. His sons grew to be hard working and productive in their community. I'm only saddened that my Grandmother Jackson did not live to see the fruit of her labor. Aunt Eunice, surrogate mother to the four youngest boys, did live to see all of them become influential men in our community. Incidentally, I have thirty-one first cousins. The next generation continued to be quite prolific as well.

"Well, Dr. Jackson, that was a generation ago. Things are different today." Yes, I understand. One of my friends is a meat cutter at a grocery store while his wife has a master's degree. They have at least twelve children (they moved away and I lost count) and live in a very modest home since she stays at home with the children. At this writing, about half of the children have graduated high school and pursued further education, contributing to our society in a positive manner. The dad's values in life are obeying God and choosing children over a culturally defined standard of living. He and his wife never felt compelled to keep up with the neighbors in their standard of living.

Many people say they could never do that. They are right because they love their stuff more than they care to obey God when He said in Genesis 2:28, "Be fruitful and multiply, and fill the earth," and more than they value children. As far as I can tell in my reading of scripture, God never rescinded His command to be fruitful and multiply. Sadly, we are more influenced by the culture around us than the clear teaching of the Word of God. Somewhere on the continuum between barrenness, which in the scripture is considered a curse, and a full quiver, which is considered a blessing, is the number of children God would give you if you were to submit to his

Lordship in that area of your life. That number is not defined in scripture, but I'm doubtful that a warrior headed into battle would want 1.87 arrows in his quiver. I'm certain he would hedge more to the "full" side — whatever that might be!

My wife and I began to notice a startling comparison between the reasons for not having children and the reasons why my abortion-minded patients wanted to have abortions. My abortion-minded patients were telling me, "Dr. Jackson, I cannot afford to have this baby. I won't be able to afford to go to college. I don't have insurance. I'll lose my job." Basically, they wanted an abortion because of financial considerations, much the same way my patients and friends limited their family size for financial reasons. That realization was quite disconcerting to my wife and me.

About that time, I read an amazing biblical account in Genesis 29:31–30:24 about Jacob, his two wives, Leah and Rachel, and the children God gave them. I encourage you to read the entire passage and meditate on it long and hard, as I did. In this passage, the two wives struggled with jealousy toward one another, mostly because of their ability or inability to bear children, and then because of their attempts to gain favor in the eyes of their husband, Jacob.

Leah was the first to conceive, and she immediately began to attribute her good fortune to the Lord, saying, "Because the Lord has seen my affliction; surely, now my husband will love me," (Genesis 29:32). She then had four sons in succession while Rachel, the wife Jacob preferred, had none. Rachel challenged Jacob saying, "Give me children, or else I die," (Genesis 30:1). Such was the intensity of her jealousy toward her sister. Can you imagine the pressure on poor Jacob?

Now notice Jacob's perceptive, albeit angry, response when he said, "Am I in the place of God, who has withheld from you the fruit of the womb?" (Genesis 30:2) Jacob recognized that ultimately God is the one who opens and closes the womb. No matter how many birth control devices my patients may use, sometimes they end up pregnant anyway, much to their dismay. No matter how much money they may spend at the fertility specialist's office, they cannot achieve a pregnancy, and then after they give up on the specialists, a year later they find themselves pregnant. Why is that? It is because God is ultimately the one who opens and closes the womb.

It is also apparent in this passage that God answers the prayers of mothers in distress. In verse 30:17, the scriptures say, "God gave heed to Leah, and she conceived..." Then in 30:22, "God remembered Rachel, and God gave heed to her and opened her womb." Never underestimate the power of pure-hearted, persistent prayers prayed within the will of God. These ladies were not really all that pure-hearted. They were filled with jealousy, yet God still answered their passionate and persistent prayers.

That means there is still hope for you and me. Some may say, "Well, all that is just coincidence." To which I would respond, "That's a lot of coincidence when you have eleven children born to eleven specific prayer requests from two women with fertility issues crying out to the Lord, 'God, give me a child.'" Sounds to me like some people just have a problem admitting to the sovereign ability of God to answer prayer and His supernatural control over the ability to produce offspring. Now put that in your pipe and smoke it!

To be honest, my wife and I had the same issues. We had three beautiful little girls. We anticipated at least having a fourth child, but what about after that? We realized the entire struggle of the Christian life was yielding control of every area of our lives up to God, right? This included our finances, our family, our future, and our reputation. We've always wanted to be that couple, but did that mean in the area of our procreativity, as well? Surely not! That notion struck fear into our hearts. I mean–He could give us ten children (based on the number of fertile years we had left when we had this discussion between us). That realization weighed heavily on our hearts. The financial implications were sobering. The health impact on my beautiful bride was a strong consideration as well.

So we began to pray — a lot! Over a long period of time, we talked to families who had lots of children; we read books, both theological and anecdotal (books that described other families' experiences). After a while we realized that it boiled down to a matter of one–faith and two–control.

Could we trust God with our procreativity like we trusted Him with our finances and our future? It would be foolish to say we trusted Him with our money, but then say,

Could we trust God with our procreativity like we trusted Him with our finances and our future?

"Oh, no, we need birth control because, God, you're not smart enough to know what is best for our family in the area of our procreativity." That's foolish and we realized it on the surface, but our hearts still struggled with it deep down. Why?

We were like everyone else — afraid. What if we had a bunch of kids and Daddy became disabled or died? This very thing happened to three of our friends who had large families (twelve, ten, and seven kids). The father in each family died suddenly, two with heart attacks and one with a blood clot to his lungs after an injury. It was a very emotional and distressing time for all the moms, the children, and friends. There was a lot of praying; God was faithful. Although huge adjustments had to be made, no one starved. Life went on. Kids graduated from high school and further education. Eventually, some married and grandchildren arrived.

We have to understand that we are fooling ourselves if we don't admit it is God "who is giving [us] power (ability) to make wealth," (Deuteronomy 8:18). When the father is available and when he is not, God is ultimately Jehovah Jireh, our Provider. In the ordinary course of events, He provides through fathers, but He is not constrained to provide for our families through fathers. Many widows and widowers live on planet Earth and God provides for them. Many of them have numerous children. I would be equally paralyzed if my wife died. I might still have an income, but I could not handle the household budget, buying groceries and clothes, or cooking meals. My children would mutiny and I would jump overboard with grief and exasperation. I can't even stand to think about it.

Here is the question: Am I going to live in fear or faith? For you see, the opposite of faith is not unbelief. The opposite of faith is fear. We manifest our faith by obedience to God even in the hard things and the socially unacceptable things — like having more than 1.8 kids.

Every time I see my friends who have more than four children, I say to them in the presence of everyone around, "Now there goes a man of real faith." When everyone looks at me with a quizzical expression, I then explain, "He has more than the standard 1.8 children. He is trusting God with His procreativity, or either his birth control doesn't work." After they finish laughing, I continue to explain, "Who is going to look after all these children if he is disabled or dead? You see, this man is really trusting in the Lord." The circle of friends usually looks at their shoes to ponder what I have said while my fertile friend walks off with his chest puffed out, thankful for the affirmation.

I have one friend who is an engineer and who has thirteen children. I love to give him that affirmation every time I see him. You know why? Because he gets what I get, "Don't you know where all these children come from? Don't you know the earth is overly populated?" I love him to death and respect him and his wife greatly. He lives a life of obedience and faith. I'm sure it is not easy for them, but I'm also sure their life is full of laughter and joy because children are a blessing and a reward. Somehow, God will honor their obedience. I like this quote from a Hungarian grandmother–"The Lord doesn't give you a little lamb without giving you a pasture for him."[2]

I had a conversation once with Rev. Flip Benham of Operation Rescue fame. He described an encounter he had in Washington, D.C., in front of television/radio reporters with several prochoice female representatives of NOW (National Organization of Women). Several prolife leaders were being interviewed by the media when a reporter asked Rev. Benham, "What makes you so confident your side will eventually win?"

Without hesitation, Rev. Benham replied, "I don't know these women personally, but let's ask them a question." Several NOW women stood opposite him while several prolife men stood beside him. Pointing to the first NOW woman, he asked, "How many children do you have?"

She replied, "One."

"How many do you have?"

"None."

"How many do you have?"

"One."

Then turning to his fellow prolife representatives, he asked, "How many children do you have?"

"Six."

"How many do you have?"

"Eight."

"How many do you have?"

"Seven."

Turning back to the reporter, Rev. Benham reported, "You understand, it is simply a matter of mathematics. In another generation, we will simply out-vote their side."

Why was Pharaoh so afraid of the Hebrew children living in the land of Goshen? Exodus 1:8 tells us the Hebrews had become too numerous. After all, they had been there for nearly 400 years. What was one thing that distinguished them from the Egyptians allowing them to outnumber the

Egyptians in population? The Egyptians practiced abortion while God's people did not.[3]

In fact, in an attempt to stem the flow, Pharaoh ordered the Hebrew midwives, Puah and Shiprah, to kill all the male Hebrew children at birth (infanticide), which they promptly refused to do since they feared God rather than the Pharaoh (Exodus 1:15-21). This is the first historical account of civil disobedience. The Bible says that God honored the Hebrew midwives for obeying God rather than the evil edict of Pharaoh. Pharaoh was enraged and determined to kill every Hebrew male child born. Sounds like modern-day China to me. America isn't far behind. About thirty percent of the abortions in America are performed on women who do not want to add to their family size.[4]

Now here is a little food for thought. What is the number one name for new baby boys in London? Don't know? Well, it's Mohammed,[5] with the Muslim population at only 12.4% of the total.[6] How can that be? It is because Muslims are not afraid to have children. It is a function of their religious belief. Muslims are fundamentally opposed to abortion and they favor childbearing. According to the Pew Research Center, the average Muslim family size worldwide is 3.1 children per family compared to the next highest religious group, Christian, at 2.7.[7] (Remember, the United States birth rate is only 1.87.) They also reported the following:

> While the world's population is projected to grow 35% in the coming decades, the number of Muslims is expected to grow at 73% — from 1.6 billion in 2010 to 2.8 billion in 2050. In 2010, Muslims made up 23.2% of the world population. Four decades later, they are expected to make up about three-in-ten of the world's people (29.7%). of the world's population [with Christians at 31.4%]. The

main reason for Islam's growth ultimately involves simple demographics. To begin with, Muslims have more children than members of the seven other major religious groups ... [plus ... they] have the youngest median age (23 in 2010) ..., seven years younger than the media age of non-Muslims (30). A larger share of Muslims will soon be at the point in their lives when people begin having children. This combined with high fertility rates, will accelerate Muslim population growth.[8]

Did you catch that phrase? It is a "simple matter of demographics"? God commanded His people to be fruitful and multiply, replenish the earth, and rule over it. Why are the false religions going to rule over the earth? It is because most Christian people are more concerned with bigger houses and retirement accounts than with trusting God in their procreativity. They are afraid to be prolific, i.e. prolife. To have a house full of children is the ultimate expression of being pro-life (whether they are your own, adopted, or foster children). A house full of children demonstrates a love for and a commitment to children. It demonstrates a willingness to die to yourself and sacrifice time/money in order to meet the needs of the children. It demonstrates a sincere desire to obey God above all else. More pointedly, it demonstrates great faith.

Where are the Christian parents who are willing to trust God with their procreativity to have as many children as God will give them and raise them in the nurture and the admonition of the Lord, teaching them to do the same until we — like the children of Israel in Egypt, who struck fear in the heart of their Egyptian oppressors by simply outnumbering them — will eventually create fear in the heart of liberals in America because our posterity outnumbers them? It is a simple matter of demographics. No, really, it is a matter of faith and obedience. The hymn writer had it right when he said, "Trust and obey, for there is no other way to be happy in Jesus but to trust and obey."[9]

One of the hardest things I have to do in my medical practice is to ask my elderly infirm patients, "Who do you have at home to help take care of you when you get sick?" It saddens me greatly when they tell me that they have no one. Most often it is because they had only one or two children or none, usually by choice, but sometimes due to fertility issues. Now, due to the vagaries of life, they have outlived their one child, or their child lives far away, or they don't get along. It's a blessing if they have a church family that looks after them, but many are not so connected.

What thrills my soul is when my patient says to me, "Doctor, don't worry about me. I have a whole passel of kids. They look after me real good. I took care of them. Now they take care of me." It almost makes me weep every time I hear my patients say that with a measure of confidence and satisfaction. Whether it's one or a half dozen, that's how it should be. Children are a reward, not a liability; blessed is the "old" man whose quiver is full of them.

So back to the struggle Mrs. Jackson and I had with our decision with birth control. While driving to Charleston, South Carolina, to a medical conference, we prayed and discussed the books we had read and our conversations with wise people in our lives. The question before us was this— were we going to trust God with this area of our lives as much as we tried to trust Him with every other area of our lives, or were we going to say we were afraid He would give us too many children? Would we consider children a blessing or a liability? Would we operate out of faith or out of fear?

We were as influenced by the culture around us as the next person, and just as concerned about what other people and family would think of us, but we finally decided we cared more about what God would think of us. As we were driving and praying, my wife suddenly opened the window and threw the birth control pills out of the window into a swamp along I-26 near Charleston. Those little fish were sterile for months!

Thus began a new adventure for the Jackson family. We began to embrace the idea of having more children. We were no longer afraid of having children. We suddenly realized that we wanted as many children as God would give us. Our whole attitude toward children had changed, even toward the ones we already had. The birth of each additional child was a cause of celebration and excitement. Our extended family, influenced by the secular culture, thought we were crazy. After each birth they said things like, "That's all now, right?"

We responded by saying, "Which one would you like to give back?" Of course, after the new baby is here they are too cute to throw back.

Our friends asked, "Are you going to have any more?"

We said, "As many as God gives us."

People ask me now, "How many children do you have?"

I respond, "Only nine. We got a late start." It's true. We got married at twenty-six and had our first child at twenty-nine. Just think what would have happened if we had started having babies earlier. It's a funny thing now that we are past the childbearing years. We loved our home full of little children to raise in the nurture and admonition of the Lord. What a joy and what a privilege! What hard work, but what a privilege! Thank the Lord we're grandparents now! Ain't life grand! At the time of this writing, we have seven grandchildren, and we've only just begun. Only four children are married – one a few months ago. Just wait until they are all married. Just call me Father Abraham!!

P.S. I have prayed since I was in college that God would have a maximum impact in my life for the kingdom of God. I always thought that would be through evangelism, teaching the Word, and disciple-making, three things I have tried to pursue faithfully. Now, after having nine children, I realize my impact on the kingdom will be greatest through the ongoing witness of my children.

My children graduated from our home school, In His Steps Academy, spiritually mature, biblically astute, and with a biblical worldview. They were way ahead of my wife and me when we entered college. They were committed to evangelism and world missions. In fact, they were ready to be world changers for the kingdom. Sure, they had some growing up to do but they were well on their way to having a significant impact for the kingdom of God.

Now I realize this is what I have been praying for myself for forty years, and suddenly I have seven of my nine children (remember two are special needs who bless others in different ways) multiplying the influence of their parents all around the globe. My oldest two daughters served as missionaries in foreign countries for several years (Venezuela and the Middle East). One of these daughters has started a Christian foster children's ministry in Alaska. The other volunteers at a crisis pregnancy center where she translated the parenting classes into Arabic for the Egyptian Coptic community.

Our third daughter is a contemporary Christian singer and has been a CPC volunteer. A fourth daughter is a part-time Christian talk show host and past event planner for a biblical worldview conference. Five children have been summer missionaries with Child Evangelism Fellowship, where they learned to share the gospel with alacrity. Our eldest son studied and served at a Christian ranch/camp for two years and has been to Guatemala on numerous mission trips, while another son finished a second summer of counseling at a Christian camp. Our youngest daughter just finished a year at the same ranch, where she spent the summer as a camp counselor. At various times they all have been Sunday School teachers, VBS workers, and choir members. My children constantly call me to tell me the latest person with whom they have shared the gospel or imparted biblical truths. The apple doesn't fall far from the tree.

I understand now that our personal legacy/impact for the kingdom of God has been multiplied tremendously through our children and even more so because of the sheer number of our children. I have no doubt the Christian influence of Robert and Carlotta Jackson will extend all over the globe because we pray every day God will raise up missionaries, pastors, Bible college professors, evangelists, Christian politicians, and homeschool moms from our posterity. (It wouldn't hurt my feelings if He sprinkled a few Christian doctors in there somewhere.)

Why does God call the children of Israel "the children of Israel"? It is because God blessed Jacob, also called Israel, with twelve male children (the twelve patriarchs) and two daughters. God blessed Jacob's father, Isaac, with two sons, Jacob and Esau. Who do we hear about the most in Scripture? Well, it is Jacob (Israel), the father of the twelve tribes of Israel, who was blessed by God with so many children and whose posterity, the Jewish people, continues to influence world events even today.

Please, hear my heart. I don't take issue at all with families who cannot bear more than one or two children due to fertility issues. I have spent many difficult hours with husbands and wives working through fertility problems. What disturbs me is Christian families that reject the opportunity to impact the world for Christ through their offspring for selfish reasons or fear.

If you are that family, my advice is try to avoid having a heart "attach." That's right–heart "attach." Don't let your heart be attached to earthly possessions so that you love your stuff more than you love the blessings that accrue to your account from having more children. Trust me, children are more of a blessing than material assets. Cultivate in your heart a biblical conviction that with Jesus there is always enough.

Jesus never runs out. He never runs dry. He is Jehovah Jireh, the Lord who provides. When we trust and obey in every area of our lives, He comes to our rescue.

Go talk to your friends who have a whole passel of kids, and they will tell you God provides. They may not be able to explain how He does it, but they pay their bills, nobody starves, and they are all pretty much happy (assuming there is no sin in the camp. Large families can experience the consequence of sin just like small families). As I said before when God gives children, He gives meat. In other words, He rewards obedience with provisions.

Am I suggesting that every couple should have as many children as they possibly can? No, not necessarily. I am suggesting that couples who are in agreement that children are a blessing and not a liability, and are willing to submit themselves to God's sovereignty over the area of their procreativity, should embrace the notion of having a large family if God so blesses. Couples who are not in agreement should pause. It would not be fair for one spouse to impose this perspective on their partner if the partner did not willingly and gladly embrace the idea of multiple children or trust in God to provide for them. That would be unwise, even foolish. I would pity the parents and the children born into such an ill-fated arrangement, destined for strife and discord.

Is a multiplicity of children purely a Christian prerogative? Of course not. The "be fruitful and multiply" mandate was recorded in Genesis long before the Christian church came into existence at Pentecost. Many families before Pentecost were blessed and favored by God by obeying the mandate. Many who yearned for children were blessed by God but were only able to have one child, i.e., Abraham and Sarah. Many non-Christian families have been blessed and favored by God and have had a quiver full even without any knowledge of this discussion. Nevertheless, they have been the beneficiaries of God's favor simply by being willing to have more than 1.8 children.

Children are a blessing in any culture. God provides for families with multiple children in any culture, Christian or not. (I will admit corrupt governments can interfere, but this book does not delve into this issue.) One doesn't have to be a Christian to benefit from obeying biblical principles. That's true for Hindus, Muslims, Buddhists, and pagan Americans. If we Christian counselors advise our lost friends to follow biblical financial principles because God will bless obedience to sound biblical advice, the same holds true for obeying God in the area of our procreativity, regardless of one's culture.

My advice to young Christian couples is to not be afraid. Don't listen to the culture around you. Trust in the Lord in every area of your life, including your procreativity. After all, it was God the Father who said, "Be fruitful and multiply and replenish the earth" (Genesis 1:28).

PSALM 127:3-5

> *Sons are a heritage from the Lord, children a
> reward from Him.*

> *Like arrows in the hands of a warrior are sons
> born in one's youth.*

> *Blessed is the man whose quiver is full of them.
> They will not be put to shame when they con-
> tend with their enemies in the gate.*

Afterword

The Next Generation

Some years ago I invited a youth group to my home for
dessert and a discussion of prolife issues. Before the discussion officially began, I sat and listened as they talked about
all manner of things. Of course, they were quite knowledge-
able concerning current movies and pop music stars. Several
of them were conversant and rather well informed about an
upcoming political race and the local candidates involved.
However, when we began our discussion of prolife issues,
they sat strangely silent. Previously, they were loud, vocal,
and opinionated. Now they had no knowledge and no opin-
ions. I was distressed, but not surprised.

After speaking to many youth groups and even adults,
I have been continually amazed at how poorly informed
Christians are on the basics of prolife thought, but then as I
told you in chapter one, so was I. Everyone has to begin their
prolife journey somewhere. I began with a little bit of prolife
education, then the Holy Spirit added conviction. Who provides the education? That is where you and I come in!

In Psalm 78:3-4 (NIV), God is teaching the importance
of instructing the next generation about "what we have heard
and known, what our fathers have told us. We will not hide
them from their children; we will tell the next generation the
praiseworthy deeds of the Lord, His power, and the wonders
He has done."

How will those coming behind us know and understand prolife principles if we don't take it upon ourselves to teach them? Will the public school teach them? Certainly not! Will Sunday School teach them? Maybe once a year on Sanctity of Human Life Sunday. How will that stand against the constant pro-death barrage from the secular media? Will you teach them at home? Yes, yes! That is your and my God-given responsibility!

> He decreed statutes for Jacob and established the law in Israel, which He commanded our forefathers to teach their children, so the next generation would know them, even the children yet to be born, and they in turn will tell their children. Then they would put their trust in God and would not forget His deeds but would keep His commands. (Psalm 78:5-7, NIV)

I heard someone say one time that Christianity is always one generation away from extinction. I disagree with that notion, because God watches jealously over His church to guard and protect her, and Jesus will present His bride to Himself "without stain or wrinkle," (Ephesians 5:27, NIV). Jesus told Peter, "And the gates of Hades shall not overpower it," (Matthew 16:18). However, I understand the concern this well-meaning person had regarding the ongoing discipling responsibility of each generation of Christians.

The same is true in the prolife movement. If we don't constantly raise up new soldiers in our ranks to replace the old warriors, our army will be depleted by attrition. Who will wave the banners? Who will speak the truth? Who will serve at the CPCs? Who will write our congressmen? Who will adopt and foster the children? It is our responsibility to "teach these children so the next generation would know them, even the children yet to be born, and they in turn will tell their children. Then they would put their trust in God ..." (Psalm 78:5-7, NIV)

Please allow me to make suggestions to make this fun and family friendly.

1) As I mentioned in a previous chapter, keep a copy of *Horton Hears a Who* for children and guests to see. It will open many opportunities for reading to small children and discussion with older children and adults. Keep the DVD and/ or book around for entertainment and discussion. Children remember these videos and the lessons they teach for a lifetime, especially if anointed with a little teaching from parents and/or grandparents. Order one from Lifecyclebooks.com.

2) Take your children and grandchildren to hear prolife speakers. As a family we have attended the annual prolife march in our state, which exposes our children and ourselves to prominent and articulate spokespersons for the prolife movement. We've participated in the annual Life Chain in October and attended our CPC banquets. I am satisfied this is why my older children consider it a natural thing to be involved in prolife ministry now.

3) Every time there is something in the newspaper about the prolife issue, discuss it at the dinner table with your children so they can become well versed at considering various nuances of the biblical, political, and legal angles. You may have to do a little research and think through the issues yourself in advance, but that is good for all of us. We should never stop learning.

4) Purchase a color monograph or CD on embryology. You don't need a medical publication unless you are a medical person. Those are expensive. It is said that the power of slavery in England was broken by the introduction of the images of slaves bound in chains. When this occurred, the emotional impact swayed the debate away from the slave traders and toward abolitionists. So, too, can we win the

debate with the truth. No one can deny the truth of a baby in a mother's womb. Show your family and friends the amazing photos of preborn babies in a mother's womb. Sincere seekers will be won over every time!

5) Ask permission to make a prolife presentation to the youth group at your church on Sanctity of Human Life Sunday if no one else is doing so. Establish your knowledge and credentials over time and then make it your business to educate the new group of teenagers every year. Expand and improve your presentation each year. Use technology to which teenagers are accustomed, i.e. Power Point, good photos. Keep up-to-date statistics. You will lose credibility with old statistics.

6) If you are confident and other people affirm you, then ask to speak to other youth groups in other churches. You are now a part of the prolife army! That is how I got started. I spoke in one church, then a youth group. Then the word got out that I could give a good presentation.

7) Keep a supply of prolife materials on hand for distribution. I use "The Questions Most People Ask About Abortion" by Melody Green. Additionally, I use "8 Week Flyer" distributed by Hayes Publishing Company, which also has ready-made teaching presentations available dealing with human life, abortion, and hard questions people ask. The best question and answer book available in my opinion, also available at Hayes Publishing, is *Why Can't We Love Them Both* by Dr. John Willke, an ob-gyn physician. I distribute these brochures when I speak in churches and at my medical office.

My calling is to educate and motivate. I educate people on the issues. I motivate them to be involved at some level in the prolife army. You can certainly do the same thing. All of these resources are currently available online.

8) If you have a personal prolife story, write it out in a brochure, get your pastor to proofread it to check your scriptures, and then distribute it like a gospel tract. You never

know how your story will impact the life of a young person in the next generation. The lessons you may have learned the hard way can make the way easier for the next generation.

9) Volunteer with your children at a local crisis pregnancy center. Talk is cheap. When your children see you actually ministering to young women in a crisis, they know you really mean what you say. When they become teenagers, it will be a natural activity for them to volunteer at the CPC, also.

10) Open your home to foster children, if you would qualify. Given the number of Christian families in most counties in our nation, no foster children should be left in the system at all. Just remember: God is enough. Make all the excuses you want to, but God is enough. These children have no one–no parents, no discipline, no Christian education, no exposure to Jesus or the church. What an awesome ministry opportunity. They may only be with you for a short time, but they will remember it for a lifetime.

Several adult young women come by my office at odd intervals to see my nurse, Mary. They hug her and talk with her for a few minutes at a time and then leave. I had no idea who these young women were for the longest time. I thought they were her extended family, which I had never met. Finally, I asked her, "Mary, who are these young ladies that come to visit you so often?" She replied, "Oh, these are my foster daughters. They just come by to say hi." Turns out, she and her husband had been foster parents to a number of children over the years. I had never known this about her. Short term ministry–long term impact!

Again:

> He declared statutes for Jacob and estab-
> lished the law in Israel, which He commanded
> our forefathers to teach our children, so the
> next generation would know them, even
> the children yet to be born, and they in turn

will tell their children. Then they would put their trust in God and would not forget His deeds but would keep His commands (Psalm 78:5-7 NIV).

As one of my good friends used to tell me, "Robert, there's nothing to it but to do it!"

"But prove yourselves doers of the word, and not merely hearers who delude themselves," (James 1:22).

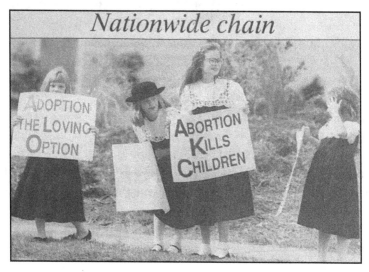

My children at the annual Life Chain

Dr. Jackson's Prayer for the Babies He Delivered

Father in Heaven,

I thank you for the safe and uncomplicated delivery of this precious little lamb. Thank you for a strong, healthy baby. What a precious gift you have given to this family. Lord, we pray this baby would be blessed with good health all the days of his life, and he would grow up to know and love you and to put you first in his life. I pray for mom and dad that they would have wisdom and discernment to raise him in the nurture and admonition of the Lord. I ask that in your time and in your way this baby would be born again into your kingdom, that you would impart to him your life. I ask, Father, in Jesus' name, that this baby would grow up to be mighty in spirit, discerning right from wrong and always choosing the good and right way. I ask, Father, that you would put in his heart a deep love for you, your Word, and your church. Lord, may 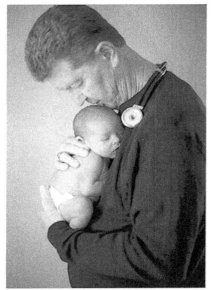 these parents raise this precious child up "in the way that he should go. So, that when he is old he may not depart from it." Lord, may this child live his life in such a way that he will always bring honor to the house of his parents and to the name of the Lord. Oh, Lord, may your hand be upon him all the days of his life. In Jesus' name, amen.

Endnotes

Chapter One

[1]C. Everett Koop, *Koop: The Memoirs of America's Family Doctor*, (New York: Random House, 1991).

[2]Thomas Pinner, SC DHEC, Divison of Biostatistics/PHSIS, pinnerta@dhec.sc.gov, October, 2016.

[3] Eric Metaxas, *Bonhoeffer: Pastor, Martyr, Prophet, Prophet, Spy— —A Righteous Gentile vs. the Third Reich*, (Nashville: Thomas Nelson, Inc. 2010). The quote is from the inside back flap of the cover. It is often attributed to Bonhoeffer but does not actually exist in any of his written works.

Chapter Two

[1]Martin Melendy, "Woman Seeks Custody of Dead Fetus," *Spartanburg Herald-Journal*, May 18, 1989, B1.

[2]Martin Melendy, "Settlements End Suits over Fatal Car Collision," *Spartanburg Herald-Journal*, March 16, 1990, C1.

[3]"Fetal Homicide State Laws," National Conference of State Legislatures, http://www.ncsl.org/research/health/fetal-homicide-state-laws.aspx, March 4, 2015, [accessed June 2015].

[4]Abby Ohlheiser, "Woman Who Cut Baby From Womb Potentially Faces More than 100 Years in Prison, DA Says," *The Washington Post*, March 27, 2015, www.washington-post.com/blogs/govbeat, [accessed June 2016].

[5]Jenna Jerman; Rachel K. Jones; and Tsuyoshi Onda, "Characteristics of U.S. Abortion Patients in 2014 and Changes Since 2008," Guttmacher Institute, May 2016, p. 6., www.guttmacher.org/sites/default/files/report_pdf/characteristics-us-abortion-patients, [accessed June 2016].

[6]Dr. and Mrs. J. C. and Barbara Wilke, *Why Can't We Love Them Both: Questions and Answers About Abortion* (Cincinnati: Hayes Publishing Co., 1997), 9.

Chapter Three

[1]Wm. Robert Johnson,Reasons Given for Having Abortions in the United States," www.johnstonsarchive.net/policy/abortion/abreasons.html, last updated January 18, 2016, [accessed June 24, 2016].

Chapter Four

[1]Mark Bradford, "New Study: Abortion after Prenatal Diagnosis of Down Syndrome Reduces Down Syndrome Community by Thirty Percent," Charlotte Lozier Institute, https://lozierinstitute.org,April 21,2015, [accessed August 10, 2016].

Chapter Five

[1]"About Abby," www.abbyjohnson.org, [accessed June 23,2016).

[2]Abby Johnson, *Unplanned: The Dramatic True Story of a Former Planned Parenthood Leader's Eye-opening Journey Across the Life Line,* (Carol Stream, Illinois: Tyndale House Publishers, Inc., 2010), 121.

[3]"About Abby."

[4]*Unplanned,* 1-7.

[5]Ibid., 124.

[6]Ibid., 146-158.

[7]"About Abby."

[8]Testimony of Norma McCorvey before the Subcommittee on the Constitution, Federalism, and Property Rights of the Senate Judiciary Committee (January 21, 1998) and before the Subcommittee on the Constitution of the Senate Judiciary Committee (June 23, 2005), www.endroe.org/mccorveytestimony.aspx and www.endroe.org/mccorvey-testimony2.aspx, [accessed June 30, 2016].

[9]Norma McCorvey, *Won by Love,* (Nashville: Thomas Nelson, Inc., 1997), 28-30.

[10]Ibid., 1-10.

[11]Ibid., 223, 228.

Chapter Six

[1]George Brown Tindall and David Emory Shi, *America: A Narrative History,* Vol. One, Seventh Edition, (New York/London: W.W. Norton & Company, 2007), 592.

[2]Harold Morris, *Twice Pardoned,* (Nashville: Thomas Nelson, Inc., 1989).

Chapter Seven

[1]Dr. Theresa Karminski Burke, "Can Relationships Survive After Abortion?" afterabortion.org/1999/can-relationships-survive-after-abortion, [accessed June, 2015].

Chapter Eight

[1]Jerry Falwell and Mel White, *If I Should Die Before I Wake*, (Nashville: Thomas Nelson, Inc., 1986).

[2]Compiled by Wm. Robert Johnston, "Historical Abortion Statistics, South Carolina (USA), last updated November 28, 2014, www.johstonsarchive.net/policy/abortion/usa/ab-usa-SC.html, [accessed July 15, 2015].

[3]Ibid.

[4]South Carolina Vital and Morbidity Statistics 2013, Vol. 1, South Carolina Department of Health and Environmental Control, Division of Biostatistics, Vital Event, Table A-2, p. 4, www.scdhec.gov/Health/docs/BiostatisticsPubs/vms2013.pdf, [accessed June 24, 2016].

[5]Ibid.

[6]Theresa Burke, Ph.D., with David C. Reardon, Ph.D., *Forbidden Grief: The Unspoken Pain of Abortion*, (Springfield: Acorn Books, 2002), xiii.

[7]"Find a Center Near You", www.sclife.org/crisis-pregnancy-centers/csu2, [accessed June 24, 2016].

[8]Amanda Coyne, "Haley has Signing Ceremony for 20-week Abortion Ban in Taylors," *The Greenville News*, www.greenvilleonline.com/story/news, [accessed August 12, 2016].

[9]"Historical Abortion Statistics"

[10]"South Carolina Abortion Clinics," www.abortion.com/abortion_ clinics_state.php?country=United%20States&state=South%20 Carolina, [accessed June 24, 2016].

Chapter Nine

[1]Theresa Burke, Ph. D. with David C. Reardon, Ph.D., *Forbidden Grief: The Unspoken Pain of Abortion*, (Springfield, Illinois: Acorn Books, 2002), 46.

[2]Ibid.

[3]Ibid.

[4]Ibid.

[5]Ibid., 47.

[6]Ibid., 48.

Chapter Ten

[1]Chandrika Narayan, "First Child Dies by Euthanasia in Belgium," September 17, 2016, http://edition.cnn. com/2016/09/17/health/belgium-minor-euthanasia, [accessed September 19, 2016].

[2]Ibid.

[3]"State-by-State Guide to Physician-Assisted Suicide," ProCon. org, last updated October 5, 2015, http://euthanasia.procon. org/view.resource.php, [accessed September 19, 2016].

[4]Dr. and Mrs. J. C. and Barbara Willke, *Why Can't We Love Them Both: Questions and Answers About Abortion* (Cincinnati: Hayes Publishing Co., 1997), 193-194 as summarized

from Fredrick Wertham's book The German Euthanasia Program, (Cincinnati: Hayes Publishing Co., 1977).

Chapter Eleven

[1]Bob Wolfe, A Drop of Life in the Sea of Time, (Minnesota: Kokoro Visions Publications, First Edition, 2011), 85.

[2]Reprint of letter to the editor by Dr. Paul E. Rockwell, "The Tiniest Human," http://www.freerepublic.com/focus/f-news/1055229/posts, [accessed June 28, 2016].

[3]Ibid.

[4]Abby Johnson, *Unplanned*, 6-7.

[5]Michael Medved, tag for *The Michael Medved Show* as heard on recorded broadcasts at http://www.michaelmedved.com and read at www.medvedhistorystore.com/complete-history-library, [accessed June 30, 2016].

[6]Mary Meehan, "Ex-Abortion Workers: Why They Quit," Article first published in *Human Life Review*, Spring/Summer 2000. Revised most recently in December 2004. http://meehanreports.com/whytheyquit.html, [accessed June 30, 2016].

[7]"Investigative Footage," www.centerformedicalprogress.org/cmp, [accessed July 1, 2016].

[8]Micaiah Bilger, "12th Video Catches Planned Parenthood Aborting Intact Late Term Babies To Sell As Parts," www.lifenews.com/2016/03/01, [accessed July 1, 2016].

[9]"Affiliate Medical Services Data," www.plannedparenthood.org/files/2114/5089/0863/2014-2015_PPFA_Annual_Report, [accessed July 1, 2016], 30.

[10]"Combined Statement of Revenue, Expenses & Changes in Net Assets: National and Affiliates," www.plannedparenthood.org/files/2114/5089/0863/2014-2015_PPFA_ Annual_Report, [accessed July 1, 2016], 33.

[11]"Abortion," www.gallup.com/poll/1576/abortion.aspx, [accessed July 1, 2016].

[12]"The RU-486 'Abortion Pill': Human Pesticide," www.texasrighttolife.com, February 24, 2015, [accessed December 13, 2016].

[13]Randall O'Bannon, Ph.D., "RU 486 Abortion Pill Marks 15th Anniversary in the US, Kills 22% of Unborn Babies Every Year," www.lifenews.com, September 23, 2015, [accessed December 13, 2016].

[14] "The RU-486 'Abortion Pill': Human Pesticide"

[15]"Induced Abortion in the United States," September, 2016 Fact Sheet, www.guttmacher.org/fact-sheet/induced-abortion-united-states, [accessed December 13, 2016].

[16]Randall O'Bannon, "While Abortions Decline, Use of RU486 Abortion Drug Up 20% in Three Years," February 12, 2014, www.lifenews.com, [accessed December 13, 2016].

[17]Steven Ertelt, "Supreme Court Allows State to Force Pro-Life Pharmacists to Sell Abortion Pills," June 28, 2016, www. lifenews.com, [accessed December 13, 2016].

[18]Dr. Seuss, *Horton Hears a Who*, (New York : Random House, 1982).

Chapter Twelve

[1]Erwin W. Lutzer, *Hitler's Cross*, (Chicago: Moody Press, 1995), 99-100.

Chapter Fourteen

[1]"The AFCARS Report", Preliminary Fiscal Year Estimates as of July 2015, www.act.hhs.gov/programs/cb, [accessed June 28, 2016], 1-2.

[2]David Platt, *Radical*, (Colorado Springs: Multnomah Books, 2010), 133.

Chapter Fifteen

[1]Dr. and Mrs. J.C. Willke, quote is from the title of the book, *Why Can't We Love Them Both: Questions and Answers About Abortion*, (Cincinnati: Hayes Publishing Company, Inc. 1997).

Chapter Sixteen

[1]Sandra Mahkorn, "Pregnancy and Sexual Assault," *The Psychological Aspects of Abortion*, eds. Mall & Watts, (Washington, D.C.: University Publications of America, 1979), 55-69.

[2]David C. Reardon, Ph. D., "Rape, Incest and Abortion: Searching Beyond the Myths," originally published in *The Post-Abortion Review 2(1)* Winter 1993, Copyright 1993 Elliot Institute, afterabortion.org/2004/rape-incest-and-abortion-searching-beyond-the-myths-3/, [accessed June 28, 2016].

[3]David C. Reardon, Julie Makimaa, and Amy Sobie, eds., *Victims and Victors: Speaking Out About their Pregnancies, Abortions and Children Resulting from Sexual Assault*, (Springfield, Illinois: Acorn Books, 2000).

[4]"Rape, Incest and Abortion: Searching Beyond the Myths"

[5]Ibid.

[6]Ibid.

[7]Dr. George Maloof, "The Consequences of Incest: Giving and Taking Life," *The Psychological Aspects of Abortion*, David Mall and Walter Watts, eds (Washington, DC: University Publications of America, 1979), 78-79, 84.

[8] "Rape, Incest and Abortion: Searching Beyond the Myths"

[9]Ibid.

[10]Ibid.

Chapter Eighteen

[1] "The World Factbook," www.cia.gov/library/publications/the-world-factbook/fields/2127.html, Fertility rates, [accessed June 28, 2016].

[2]Mary Pride, *The Way Home Beyond Feminism Back to Reality*, (Wheaton, Illinois: Crossway Books, 1985), 64.

[3]"Ancient Egyptian Facts," http://www.ancientegyptian-facts.com/ancient-egypt-abortion.html, [accessed June 28, 2016].

[4] Lawrence B. Finer, Lori F. Frohwirth, Lindsay A. Dauphinee, Susheela Singh and Ann M. Moore, "Reasons U.S. Women Have Abortions: Quantitative and Qualitative Perspectives," *Perspectives an Sexual and Reproductive Health*, 2005, 37(3), 113.

[5]Ann Davis, "Revealed: The Most Popular Names for Babies in London; Official Data Reveals the Most Popular Names for Babies Across the UK," www.standard.co.uk/news/london/revealed-the-most-popular-name-for-baby-boys-in-lon-

don-according-to-official-date-a2871406.html, August 17, 2015, [accessed August 11, 2016]

6"Religion in England and Wales 2011," http://www.ons.gov.uk/peoplepopulationandcommunity/culturalidentity/religion/articles/religioninenglandandwales2011/2012-12-11, December 11, 2012, [accessed August 11, 2016]

7Michael Lipka and Conrad Hackett, "Why Muslims are the World's Fastest-growing Religious Group," April 23, 2015, http://www.pewresearch.org/fact-tank/2015/04/23/why-muslims-are-the-worlds-fastest-growing-religious-group, [accessed August 12, 2015]

8Ibid.

9John H. Sammis, "Trust and Obey," The Baptist Hymnal, (Nashville: Convention Press, 1991), 447.

CPSIA information can be obtained
at www.ICGtesting.com
Printed in the USA
JSHW030725161222
34910JS00011B/8